Medical Musings

Medical Musings

Second Edition

Robert T. Sataloff, M.D., D.M.A., F.A.C.S.

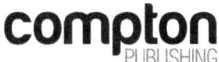

This edition first published 2019 © 2019 by Compton Publishing Ltd.

Registered office: Compton Publishing Ltd, 30 St. Giles', Oxford, OX1 3LE, UKRegistered company number: 07831037

Editorial offices: 35 East Street, Braunton, EX33 2EA, UKWeb: www.comptonpublishing.co.uk

The right of the authors to be identified as the authors of this work has been asserted in accordance with the UK Copyright, Designs and Patents Act 1988.

All rights reserved. No part of this publication may be reproduced, stored in a retrieval system, or transmitted, in any form or by any means, electronic, mechanical, photocopying, recording or otherwise, except as permitted by the UK Copyright, Designs and Patents Act 1988, without the prior permission of the publisher.

Trademarks: Designations used by companies to distinguish their products are often claimed as trademarks. Any brand names and product names used in this book are trade names, service marks, trademarks or registered trademarks of their respective owners. The publisher is not associated with any product or vendor mentioned in this book.

Disclaimer: This book is designed to provide helpful information on the subject discussed. This book is not meant to be used, nor should it be used, to diagnose or treat any medical condition. For diagnosis or treatment of any medical condition, consult your own physician. The publisher and author are not responsible for any specific medical condition that may require medical supervision and are not liable for any damages or negative consequences to any person reading or following the information in this book. References are provided for informational purposes only and do not constitute endorsement of any product, website, or other source.

Permissions: Where necessary, the publisher and author(s) have made every attempt to contact copyright owners and clear permissions for copyrighted materials. In the event that this has not been possible, the publisher invites the copyright owner to contact them so that the necessary acknowledgments can be made.

ISBN 978-1-909082-63-2

A catalogue record for this book is available from the British Library.

Cover design: David Siddall, http://www.davidsiddall.com

Set in Caslon Pro by Kerrypress Ltd, St Albans

1   2019

Contents

Acknowledgements ix
List of contributors xi
Preface xiii

Part I: Education 1

1. 'Full-time' faculty: An evolving construct? 3
2. Academic medicine: A training gap 6
3. The academic practice of medicine 9
4. Resident duty hours: Concerns and consequences 19
5. Consistency of medical student education: Otolaryngology as a model for medical student subspecialty training 25
6. Fellowship training in otolaryngology 29
7. Interdisciplinary opportunities for creativity in medicine 32
8. Physicians studying voice and the arts 36
9. Arts medicine: An interdisciplinary paradigm 40
10. Education in laryngology: Rising to old challenges 43
11. World Voice Day 57
12. The otolaryngology residency application problem 60
13. Interviews: Less helpful than we think, or harmful 65
14. Hiring young doctors: What physicians should know about changes in the medical school curriculum 68

Part II: Research — 72

15. HIPAA: An impediment to research — 74
16. Evidence-based medicine — 78
17. Evidence-based medicine: Yet more concerns — 81
18. Clinical trials: The case for registration — 84
19. Drug development research: The process — 87
20. Understanding the regulation of pharmaceutical drug promotion — 90
21. Quality of reporting in randomized trials — 94
22. Human subject research or quality improvement project? — 96
23. Practice parameters and clinical practice guidelines: Science, politics, and problems — 99
24. Centralized Otolaryngology Research Efforts (CORE) grants — 103
25. Reg-ent: An invaluable new offering from the American Academy of Otolaryngology-Head and Neck Surgery — 105
26. Access to quaternary care — 108
27. Data Scientists: They know what we don't know that we don't know about Big Data — 111

Part III: Publication — 116

28. Peer review: Universal, but valid? — 118
29. The editorial process: Resident and graduate student education and participation — 123
30. Correcting the medical literature: Ethics and policy — 127
31. Publication as a teaching tool — 130
32. Journal ethics: Let the reader beware — 133
33. Case reports in medicine — 135

Part IV: Politics — 137

34. Healthcare for the uninsured: A simpler, cheaper, faster, better solution — 139
35. Undermining market forces: A fundamental flaw in American healthcare — 144
36. Healthcare system failure: A planned strategy? — 148
37. Price controls in medical practice — 152
38. Tort reform: Federal impetus for change — 155
39. The Board of Directors — 159
40. Politics: Getting involved — 163
41. Politics: Be part of it — 167
42. Establishing federal laws — 169
43. New problems in the scope-of-practice controversy — 172

Part V: Clinical Practice — 175

44. Was that my doctor? — 177
45. Women in Otolaryngology–Head and Neck Surgery — 179
46. Disruptive physicians: Sound more familiar than you thought? — 183
47. Hearing loss: Economic impact — 186
48. Evaluating occupational hearing loss: The value of the AMA's Guides to the Evaluation of Permanent Impairment — 189
49. Emotional intelligence and physician wellness — 194
50. Shoulder injuries related to vaccine administration (SIRVA): A potential problem for all physicians — 197
51. Part-time physicians — 200
52. Adverse surgical events: Effects on the surgeon — 204
53. Geriatric surgery — 207
54. Telemedicine — 211
55. The aging physician and surgeon — 218

Part VI: Miscellaneous Musings — 247

56. Teamwork — 249
57. Longevity: The disposable soma? — 252
58. The physician as an expert witness — 255
59. Unethical Surgery — 258
60. Physicians and retirement — 261

About the Author — 266
Index — 268

Acknowledgements

Compton Publishing wishes to thank the following publishers who gave their kind permission to modify and reproduce their copyrighted materials in this book: Vendome Group, LLC, for materials from *Ear, Nose & Throat Journal* (http://www.entjournal.com); SAGE Publications, Inc., for material published in *Annals of Otology, Rhinology & Laryngology* (http://www.annals.com); and Plural Publishing, Inc., for material published in *Professional Voice: The Science and Art of Clinical Care*, Fourth Edition, and *Diagnosis and Treatment of Voice Disorders*, Fourth Edition.

The author is indebted to Mary Hawkshaw, R.N., B.S.N., CORLN, for her invaluable help in preparing and critiquing these manuscripts, Debbie Westergon for her expert manuscript processing, and Linda Zinn for her numerous excellent editorial suggestions in the editorials in *Ear, Nose & Throat Journal* from which many of these chapters were modified.

Contributors

Shyam K. Akula, M.D.-Ph.D.
Student, Harvard-MIT M.D.-Ph.D. Program; Harvard Stem Cell Institute M.D-Ph.D. Fellow, Boston, MA

Mary J. Hawkshaw, R.N., B.S.N., CORLN
Research Professor, Department of Otolaryngology–Head and Neck Surgery, Drexel University College of Medicine, Philadelphia, Pennsylvania

Natalie A. Krane, M.D.
Department of Otolaryngology–Head and Neck Surgery, Oregon Health & Science University, Portland, Oregon

Joshua Kutinsky, J.D., Psy.D.
Institute of Graduate Clinical Psychology, Widener University, Chester, Pennsylvania ; Aetna Life Insurance Company, Blue Bell, Pennsylvania

Edward Maitz, Ph.D.
Assistant Professor, Department of Otolaryngology–Head and Neck Surgery, Drexel University College of Medicine, Philadelphia, Pennsylvania

John S. Rubin, M.D., F.A.C.S., F.R.C.S.
Consultant Otolaryngologist, Royal National Throat, Nose and Ear Hospital; Honorary Consultant Otolaryngologist, National Hospital for Neurology and Neurosurgery, University College London Hospitals NHS Trust; Honorary Visiting Professor, School of Health Sciences, City University of London; Honorary Senior Lecturer, Department of Surgery, University College London

Preface

This collection of publications excludes all of my 'scientific' writings. It includes only 'opinion pieces', many of which are modified from editorials that I wrote for *Ear, Nose & Throat Journal*. It is offered to provide perspectives on education, publication, health care delivery, and other topics relevant to leadership in medicine, and more importantly to inspire thought and provoke debate.

I am indebted to Vendome Publishers for permission to modify and republish material that appeared in *Ear, Nose & Throat Journal*, which constitutes all but three of the chapters in this book; to SAGE Publications, Inc. and the *Annals of Otology, Rhinology & Laryngology*, for permission to republish 'Education in laryngology: Rising to old challenges'; and, to Plural Publishing, Inc., for permission to republish 'Physicians Studying Voice and the Arts' and 'Telemedicine'. Hopefully, this book will serve as a convenient, updated collection for colleagues who read *Ear, Nose & Throat Journal* and the other publications from which these chapters were derived, and a resource of new materials for those who do not.

If this collection leads to writing of editorials and opinion pieces by those who read these musings (whether they agree or disagree with the opinions expressed herein), then I will consider this small book a success.

Robert T. Sataloff, M.D., D.M.A., F.A.C.S.
Professor and Chairman, Department of Otolaryngology–Head and Neck Surgery and Senior Associate Dean for Clinical Academic Specialties Drexel University College of Medicine

Part I: Education

1. Full-time faculty: An evolving construct?

In another publication, I reviewed *The Academic Practice of Otolaryngology*.[1] That article makes the case that academic practice is a state of mind, not a source of employment. It is possible for all of us to remain academically and intellectually vital throughout our careers, regardless of whether we are employed by universities or even have university affiliation. Throughout the history of medicine, many of our most important innovations and discoveries were made by private practitioners. Nevertheless, during the last few decades, there has been a shift of academically active physicians toward a university employment model, partly because of changes in the economics of medical practice. Previously, even many 'full-time' academicians were really geographic full-time physicians who practiced at a university but whose economics depended almost entirely on a private-practice model. This included even department chairs at venerable institutions such as the University of Michigan. This model was successful partly because of the altruistic culture of volunteer faculty and the graciousness with which they were integrated into teaching programs. Integration of volunteer faculty from numerous practices also enhanced resident training through more diverse exposure than is generally available through a single group, even many academic departments.

Although that model has been virtually abandoned recently at many institutions, it has not been forgotten; and it may warrant reconsideration. Institutions throughout the United States and elsewhere are struggling with the economic pressures of healthcare delivery and education. While there was a time when it was possible to provide substantial support to medical schools through excess income from physician faculty, such heady days are gone in most places. Recently, most academic institutions in the United States have responded to such pressures by trying to minimize or eliminate the role of volunteer faculty in order to maximize the practice plan's market share, influencing clinicians to either leave universities or become full-time, salaried employees. Although this strategy has worked at some institutions, it has resulted in 'red ink' for more than a few practice plans, particularly in some of the nonsurgical disciplines. Moreover, it has forced many experienced clinicians and teachers to abandon institutions whose reputations they helped establish, often taking their patients and prestige with them. This situation naturally leads one to wonder whether there is a sensible alternative to the current trend toward 'full-time or no-time' academic practice.

One solution may be a shift back toward the model that worked so well throughout the first three-quarters of the 20th century. Many of us over 50, and most physicians over 70, were trained by dedicated clinical teachers and scientists who were committed to resident and medical student education, who amassed an impressive record of advances in the field and who did all their teaching on a volunteer or 'geographic full-time' basis. Most paid no 'dean's tax', but they also charged institutions little or nothing.

They were responsible for their own economic success or failure and never generated any red ink for an institution. While changes in the economics of private practice have made this model more challenging, the trend toward minimizing or abandoning its potential contribution to academic programs does not seem to be the most sensible solution. It is time for us to reassess the structure of our academic faculties and to reconsider models that combine full-time, salaried clinical and research faculty (perhaps in somewhat smaller numbers) more effectively with volunteer faculty whose academic status and title are determined by their academic performance, rather than by the source of their income.

In these days of limited resources, it makes little sense to squander clinical and academic expertise that used to be incorporated into our educational programs at little or no cost to academic institutions. It was the model that got us where we are. While the pendulum may never swing back to a complete dependence on this model (and probably should not), it is time to consider whether the pendulum has swung too far toward the other extreme and to open our minds and our institutions to a structure that incorporates the best of both approaches to medical education.

References

1. Sataloff RT. The academic practice of otolaryngology: Philosophical and practical perspectives. *Ann Otol Rhinol Laryngol* 2006;115:403–7.

Reprinted with modifications by permission of Vendome Group from:
Sataloff RT. 'Full-time' faculty: An evolving construct. *ENT J* 2006

2. Academic medicine: A training gap

Following receipt of a Doctorate of Medicine, most physicians pursue postdoctoral training. This training is usually 4 to 8 years in duration. In most cases, it involves educational tasks with supervision for approximately 80 hours per week, didactic lectures averaging 3 to 6 hours per week (more in some programs), various intensive special courses, nationally standardized 'in-service examinations' given annually, and a nationally standardized board examination.

Exceptional residents have found time to publish and pursue scholarly activities in addition to fulfilling other residency requirements. Following residency, at least some of the best and brightest trainees pursue careers in academic medicine, perhaps after fellowship training. However, do our residency programs, train people adequately for academic careers? In this writer's opinion, the answer is no.

Ideally, a skilled career academic physician should have a substantial knowledge base regarding teaching, evaluation, organizations involved in medical education and certification, and many other topics. At present, such special information is learned 'on the job'. This takes several years and commonly results in misconceptions, misinformation and knowledge gaps among clinical faculty nationwide.

To improve the quality of our educators, it seems worthwhile to try to identify the gaps in our present education system and develop strategies to fill them. Ultimately, it would be ideal to include additional training in education and leadership within our residency curriculum. An alternative would be the creation of new educational programs to address this problem. For example, a Master of Science in academic medicine has been proposed at Drexel University College of Medicine (disclosure: as a member of the faculty, I have an interest in this graduate education program). A portion of the reasoning behind this program and its content is presented in this chapter to initiate broader discussion about what we should be teaching our teachers, and how we might do so.

The MS in academic medicine was designed for residents and faculty (especially young faculty) currently in training or practice, and it is intended to provide - in a convenient, organized fashion - information valuable in an academic setting. Details of this 35-credit-hour program will not be reviewed in this chapter. Summarizing the content of two components (core knowledge and research education) should help the reader understand how academic training might help prepare physicians better for academic careers than most residencies and fellowships do now.

One solution to the perceived problem of inadequate preparation for academic practice was the creation of a two-semester didactic course, entitled Academic Medicine: Core Knowledge. This course provides lectures, supplemented by interactive training and targeted projects. It includes overviews of topics that generally are not addressed in detail during residency training, but are important to academicians. These are intended to at least give students an introduction to selected subjects so that the students understand the scope of the topic and have some grasp of what they do not know.

Topics in the two-semester Core Knowledge course include, among others, principles of leadership; principles of education; techniques of assessment and evaluation; core competencies; professionalism; bioethics; politics and organized medicine; accrediting organizations (Association of American Medical Colleges, Accreditation Council for Graduate Medical Education, the Joint Commission, etc.); legal issues in academic medicine; CV preparation; entrepreneurship; biotechnology; medical writing; medical editing; grant writing; funding sources (federal, private, and industrial); academic health center management (how to prepare a business proposal to support a capital budget request, for example); public speaking; and human research practices and regulations. These and numerous other topics included in the curriculum provide information and vocabulary that make us more effective in an academic setting but that many of us do not acquire during residency. Hopefully, we will in the future.

Research is important in academic practice, of course, but teaching research may be even more important to a career medical educator. Some residency programs have excellent systems for teaching and supervising resident research, but many do not. Too often, residents' research training has involved coming up with an idea, proposing it to an attending, and being told 'that is a good idea.' The research requirement in our academic medicine Masters program is designed not so much to result in great research (although acceptance for publication in a peer-reviewed journal is required) but, rather, to expose the trainee to a systematic process for pursuing and teaching research.

The required research project involves a thesis committee with at least one basic scientist; presentation of a proposal; revision of the proposal; preparation with mentorship of the committee before beginning the research, including consultation with a statistician; completion of a literature review and other requirements; progress reports to the committee; and thesis defense. This rigorous research training model is used routinely by our colleagues in the basic sciences. It seems clear that academic clinicians should advocate a rigorous training process for research preparation, execution, and evaluation. This tradition of systematic preparation and evaluation should be present in all of our training programs, not just some of the 'better' ones.

Residency and fellowship training are excellent in many ways, but we should always be looking for opportunities to improve. Whether we choose to educate our future academic leaders in the long run by incorporating education and leadership training into all residency curricula, through national Academy courses, or through graduate programs, we should be thinking and talking about strategies to improve the academic knowledge and skills of current and future generations of physician educators.

Reprinted with modifications by permission of Vendome Group from:
    Sataloff RT. Academic medicine: A training group. *ENT J* 2012;91(8):306–8.

3. The academic practice of medicine

The practical exigencies of medical practice in the 21st century have changed the way many physicians view medicine. Conversations among physicians used to center on interesting cases and scientific concepts. Now, they focus more often on managed care, shrinking resources, electronic medical records and other issues that have not been central concerns among physicians traditionally. Since we lead by example, this change in focus has certainly affected the thinking of our medical students, residents and fellows. While it is clear that we need to be more diligent than we were in past years about the business and political aspects of medical practice and health care delivery, we must be careful also not to lose sight of the altruistic propensities that attracted most of us to medicine. Although our first obligation is to provide outstanding medical care, all physicians also should accept an obligation to nurture an academic component within our practices, and to prevent ourselves from being consumed exclusively by daily clinical and business demands. All of us can spend eighteen hours a day, seven days a week, delivering direct patient care. However, in doing so, are we making the best possible contribution to our patients, community and profession? If we set aside even one-half day, or one day per week for reading, writing for publication, lecturing, creative thinking about clinical issues, and research, we can learn and contribute much; and such creative thinking keeps us enthusiastic and intellectually sharp as clinicians.

Academic practice does not necessarily mean university employment or even university affiliation, although active involvement in formal academic medicine and teaching is invaluable to the field and the individual practitioner; and it should be encouraged. However, even practitioners in locations remote from medical centers now have easy access to colleagues and new information through electronic and other media. Hence, it is easier than ever before not only to remain current with new developments, but also to contribute to our evolving specialty through research and publications.

Research

What is research, and why should we, as clinicians, care? Every physician sees patients that he or she cannot cure or even help much, beyond providing the comfort of personal support and hope. Faced with this common situation, we can either be satisfied, say to ourselves 'Well, I can't help everybody' and accept our limitations, or we can remain steadfastly dissatisfied with the limitations of our knowledge. In this author's opinion, the latter choice is essential if we are to help as many people as possible throughout our careers, and if we are to advance the field of medicine. If we choose to be dissatisfied with our limitations and to do something about them, then we must ask the question 'What do I need to know in order to be able to help the next person with the same problem?' Defining that question and working toward its answer is called research. Investigations may be clinical or bench research. Initially, the notion of bench research may seem a bit daunting especially in areas remote from university medical centers. However, most hospital pathology departments and many college science departments have a surprising wealth of equipment, expertise, and laboratory facilities; and many are very anxious to collaborate with physicians in research. In fact, the usual limitation in such efforts is the physician's time; and that is under our control.

Traditionally, full-time, university-based clinicians have been provided with the support and resources necessary to facilitate academic endeavors including research. However, in recent years even university-based physicians have felt economic pressures that may limit research; and faculty have had to put forth extra effort to protect research time and resources. Yet, research is still practical for academicians and even for independent practitioners. Most of us have many questions every day. If we keep in mind a few basic principles, the concept of research does not seem so overwhelming. First, we need to remember the KISS principle. This acronym stands for 'keep it simple, stupid' and it is a fundamental wisdom in every research laboratory. For us, it means that before embarking on a project, we need to devote time and thought to defining a question that can be answered, and that will get us closer to solving a problem worthy of our time. Unfortunately, by the end of a busy day, we have forgotten most of them. To prevent the loss of ideas, keep a list. The list may be several pages long and should include every idea that crosses our mind for a possible paper or research project. We should get in the habit of jotting down or dictating such ideas whenever we have them and keeping an updated list of 'research and projects to do'.

Second, we should build a research team. Although this might appear easier in a university setting, it is possible in any office; and sometimes it is even easier in a private practice unencumbered by university bureaucracy. In addition to the physician, in, say, an ENT team there might be included a specialist or interested nurse, physician assistant, medical assistant, audiologist, speech-language pathologist, physical therapist, medical librarian, consulting physician, medical student, nursing student, hospital intern, nearby-college faculty member or graduate student, research scientist, statistician, spouse or other person. The team should definitely include someone with knowledge of statistics and research design. There is a statistician in most communities that have even a modest-sized hospital or college. When no one is available locally, such collaboration can be obtained easily through a college or medical center anywhere. Usually, it is easiest to try first either the nearest medical center or the one at which the physician trained, where he or she is likely to have contacts already. It is highly advisable to consult with a statistician before beginning any project, in order to refine research design and avoid having to repeat analyses or discard data. Similar constructive criticism may be offered also by an Institutional Review Board (IRB). IRB review and approval are required for any research involving human subjects, if any portion of the research is being done for research purposes only (as opposed to necessary clinical care that would be provided anyway), utilizes confidential health information, or if the research uses experimental devices or drugs. It is often wise to consult an IRB even if IRB approval may not be mandatory, not only to solicit constructive suggestions from the IRB, but also because IRB approval, or a written opinion stating that IRB approval is unnecessary, is prudent from a medical legal and ethical standpoint and may be required by some journals.

Starting research projects may require little more than a burst of enthusiasm; but completing them productively can be challenging. Finishing research projects and publications is made easier by following a systematic approach. Steps one and two are recognizing a problem and defining the question to be studied, as noted above. Step three is a literature review. This should be thorough and scholarly, and should include not only new literature, but also review of historical literature, much of which was written prior to the 1960s and might not be listed in computer databases. Books and book chapters are also generally not indexed in medical computer databases (yet). Indexed new literature from many journals is readily accessible over the Internet.

However, it should be remembered that there are many thousands of medical journals that are not listed in Index Medicus or by the Institute for Scientific Information (ISI) and which, like older literature, may not be found through computer searches alone. This problem can be solved by one or more of the team going to a good medical library. Alternatively, it is possible to retain the services of a medical librarian, graduate student, medical student, or resident at a medical center. Medical librarians are expert at finding obscure references. Their services are well worth the cost of their time and the photocopying charges for the literature they find. If the physician or his/her representative does the library research without a consulting librarian, it is helpful to assess all of the current literature first, and to study the bibliographies for leads to unindexed literature of interest.

The next step is to review the literature thoroughly and to summarize it. Certainly, the lead physician will need to read all of the literature; but the initial review and summary can be done nicely by allied health colleagues, or anyone else with basic knowledge of the field and training sufficient to write a high school term paper. Colleagues who contribute substantively by participating in research preparation and publications in this fashion should be included as co-authors.

Based upon what was learned from the literature, the original question being studied might need to be redefined. At this point, consultation with a statistician should be obtained before finalizing the clinical or basic study design. It is also a good idea at this point to talk with a mentor, for instance, a former professor who is familiar with the subject matter. Often, such experts are aware of unpublished work, previous failed efforts, or research in progress elsewhere that may affect the research plan. Details of carrying out the research depend upon the nature of the project and will not be reviewed in detail in this publication. Once the project is completed and the data are analyzed, it is important to 'go the last mile' and write a manuscript for publication.

Publishing

If journals contained only top-quality, prospective research data, we would have far fewer journals than we do. There are many good reasons to publish and many venues in which one can publish. From the physician's standpoint, very few activities teach us more than we learn from writing a paper, chapter, or book. The process helps us organize what we know and identify knowledge gaps. Hence, it is not only educational and intellectually stimulating, but also an invaluable asset to our clinical practices. There are many other good reasons to write and publish. For example, if a physician needs to spend several hours in the library or on the Internet learning about a clinical entity, it is worth writing a review article (and possibly case series) summarizing all available information, so that the next physician interested in this problem only needs to read one, definitive article.

Physicians (in residency and thereafter) often spend many hours preparing excellent lectures to be presented at grand rounds, or in other venues. These lectures are often comprehensive summaries worthy of publication either in the physician's specialty literature, or in more general medical literature for educational purposes. Often all that is required is to record and transcribe the lecture and add references. Yet, too many physicians neglect this last step and do not optimize their hours spent in preparation.

Case reports have value when they serve as the inspiration for a scholarly review synthesizing disparate literature, report the findings and course of a rare clinical entity, and/or describe novel treatment approaches and their outcomes. They are also valuable when they discuss complications and their management which many physicians are reluctant to report, but which may have enormous educational value. It is difficult to get case reports published in many mainstream medical journals, and they often are relegated to case report journals (particularly open access case report journals). However, it often is relatively easy to convert a case report to a case series. This can be done by searching medical records from one's practice, hospital and affiliated institutions. This search may reveal another 20 or 30 patients with the same condition encountered over the previous decade, or earlier. Including these patients not only makes the paper more valuable and might reveal previously unrecognized trends that are clinically valuable, but it also changes the paper from a case report to a more meaningful case series that is much more likely to be published. Many physicians also are reluctant to publish retractions correcting or modifying their previously-published but erroneous opinions. Yet, correcting the literature is especially important and should be considered a scientific and ethical priority. Reports of large clinical series are also often instructive. Once again, such information does not require that a practitioner be located at a major university medical center. Innumerable large series of great academic importance have emanated from private practitioners throughout the history of medicine.

Obviously, the promulgation of new ideas, new discoveries, and new surgical procedures also warrants publication. However, it is important to remember that every publication does not need to win a Nobel Prize. In fact, when we look back on what we read during residency, most of the publications in our literature are not of intimidating brilliance. Sharing our concepts, insights and experience is intrinsically valuable to our colleagues and our field; and most substantial contributions are built one small step at a time.

When planning to publish, we must choose the best form. Alternatives include articles, book chapters, books, abstracts, posters, audio or video tapes, CD-ROM and other media. The choice depends upon the nature of the subject, the facilities at our disposal (such as computer expertise), and the audience we wish to reach. Most of the journals we read are peer-reviewed scientific medical journals. In many ways, they provide the best source of information for us, because the review process tries to provide reasonable assurance of reliability, validity and relevance. Input from expert reviewers can be invaluable in helping to recognize and correct weaknesses in a paper before it is published. Rather than being offended by insightful criticism, authors should appreciate the assistance of an editorial board in helping to ensure that each paper is as good as is possible and that potentially misleading or embarrassing oversights are not perpetuated in print. It is also important to recognize that although scholarly reviews are usually correct, there are exceptions. Editors make great efforts to assign manuscripts to appropriate reviewers; and most reviewers request reassignments of manuscripts that they do not feel qualified to review; but the system is not perfect. On those rare occasions when an author feels certain that the reviewer did not understand the subject or really missed the point, it is appropriate to call the matter to the attention of the Editor-in-Chief and request reconsideration by another reviewer. In the author's experience writing more than 1,000 publications, this has only happened once, although disagreement with one or two suggestions in a lengthy review is not uncommon. The choice of a publication venue also deserves contemplation and depends largely on four questions:

1. Will it be presented?
2. Why was it written?
3. Who should read it?
4. Who may accept it?

If the material will be presented at a national or international meeting, submission to a journal affiliated with the meeting may be mandatory. For example, *Laryngoscope* has right of first refusal for materials presented at meetings of the Triological Society; and there are many similar affiliations. If the journal choice is not predetermined by virtue of presentation of the paper at a meeting, then the author needs to answer the remaining three questions. If the article was written to provide specialists in his/her own discipline with new information, then clearly it belongs in a specialty journal in that field. However, if it is an article that provides no new information, it is not likely to get accepted by one of the specialty's major journals. Nevertheless, it may have value as a book chapter (print or online) or as a review article in a related field.

For an otolaryngologist, for example, such fields might include pediatrics, internal medicine, neurology, general surgery, pulmonology, gastroenterology, neurosurgery, or family medicine.

If the article is a relatively erudite treatise written primarily for fellow subspecialists, it may be most appropriate for one of more prestigious specialty journals. Yet, it should be remembered that some of these journals have small circulations between 1,000 and 6,000. If the article has practical value for a larger group of physicians (e.g. general otolaryngologists as opposed to otologists, or general internists as opposed to just pulmonologists or cardiologists), it may be better to have it published in a less 'prestigious' journal, with a larger circulation. If the article is written as a review to educate family practitioners and internists, it may be best to consider a non-peer reviewed, controlled circulation journal, some of which have circulations of over 100,000. Providing information to such colleagues is often as valuable as writing for specialists in our own field. Obviously, if the article is of sufficient merit to be acceptable to a journal that is peer reviewed, prestigious and has a large circulation. such as *Journal of the American Medical Association (JAMA)*, that is preferable; but failure to meet that standard does not mean that the article is not worth publishing. The author should also consider any time pressure related to publication and should not hesitate to make journal editors aware of special situations. If the article includes time-sensitive data or materials that will create important, immediate changes in the standard of care, it is not unreasonable to notify the editor of the journal and request expedited review and publication. Many articles spend three months or more in the review process and a year thereafter before they appear in print. Such requests are not appropriate for routine papers or most review articles.

Most of our better-known, peer-reviewed journals are indexed by Index Medicus, Scopus and/or the Institute for Scientific Information (ISI), which means that people who rely on computers will be able to locate articles from those journals when they enter key words relevant to the subject. This highlights the need for care in selecting key words for each of our manuscripts, since they will determine whether colleagues ever find our work! Yet, authors should be aware that only a small percentage of medical and scientific journals are indexed, and the fact that a journal is well-known and peer-reviewed does not necessarily mean that it is listed in Index Medicus or ISI and available through related databases. The indexing process involves economic considerations, and perhaps even 'political' factors; and funds permit the indexing by Index Medicus of only about 5,000 of the approximately 30,000 medical journals currently in print. Few journals are indexed within their first five years of existence. This does not mean that authors should not support new scholarly journals by contributing articles; but they should consider indexing as one factor in selecting a journal and should be aware of alternate ways to assure that articles that are published in such journals are eventually included in the major computer databases.

The issue of duplicate publication is interesting, and not as clear-cut as it might appear. Duplicate publication does not necessarily mean repeating verbatim the same material, but rather publishing substantial portions or concepts that were published previously by the same author, especially if the original publication is not referenced. It may also include publishing different portions of the same research in separate articles (so-called 'salami slicing'), in some cases. Attention must be paid to copyright law and to academic ethics, of course; but one can argue reasonably that the appropriateness of duplicate publication is affected by the material, and the reason for publication. If an article is presenting new research data, these data should be published once in a peer-reviewed journal. Still, they may be included (with appropriate citation and, if necessary, a permission) in later review articles or book chapters. If authors are publishing largely to enhance their chances for academic promotion, then publishing the same article two or three times with a slightly different title is unethical; and such behavior has led, in part, to the current 'hard line' against duplicate publication. However, if an author's primary motivation is to educate colleagues and improve patient care, then it may be reasonable to argue that anything worth publishing once, is worth publishing at least twice. As a journal Editor-in-Chief, this author recognizes that such a statement is heresy. Nevertheless, he also realizes that the practice is not only common, but also sometimes useful. Many people reuse portions of their best articles as book chapters, tutorial review articles, or as slightly revised articles with a few more cases or subjects, published in a journal that reaches a different readership from that of the first publication. If the reuse is made clear to the new journal, if the original works are cited in the newer publications and, as stated, if appropriate acknowledgments are given and copyright laws are obeyed, then the only consequence of this practice may be that more people read the material and learn. These opinions are controversial, but if we can agree that publication should serve to enhance and educate, then this author would argue that the subject of 'duplication publication' deserves thoughtful and ongoing reconsideration.

Another excellent way to stay active academically is to become involved with journal peer-review. Peer-review is a process for selecting papers for publication based on merit, as determined by 'experts' in their respective field(s). Medical journal editors, editorial boards and reviewers receive large numbers of submissions. Journals try to select papers that are honest, valid and free of inappropriate bias.

There are several techniques for peer-review. The most common is single-blind, during which reviewers know who the authors are, but reviewers remain anonymous. In double-blind review, both the reviewers and authors are anonymous. However, from a practical standpoint, experienced reviewers often infer authorship based on content, language and citations. In open reviews, the identity of the authors and the reviewers is known to both parties. Post-publication review is a newer approach. Essentially, articles are published as submitted. Reviews and critiques are published either with or following the published article. Papers published for post-publication review usually are published online.

Excellent peer-reviewed journals have a bias toward evidence-based research. This has been true particularly in the 21st century. There is wide belief that high-level evidence-based research (such as double-blind, prospective research) is more likely to be valid; although there is certainly also value in observational studies and reports by experts with vast experience who present clinical data. Interestingly, there is an astonishing paucity of evidence-based data supporting the value of the peer-review process. Most of the credible publications on peer-review are derived from surveys distributed by the Publishing Research Consortium.[1,2]

One does not need to be a university professor to participate as a reviewer for excellent peer-reviewed journal. Editors always welcome participation by interested colleagues who are willing to prepare insightful reviews expeditiously. Private practitioners should not hesitate to contact journal editors and express an interest in reviewing articles, providing a CV and specifying specialty or subspecialty topics on which the reviewer is comfortable offering opinions.

Teaching

Every physician has opportunities to teach. In practice settings remote from a medical school, the 'students' may be referring physicians, interns, ancillary medical personnel, office staff (colleagues often like to know about the subjects they are transcribing or the surgery they schedule), or patients. Teaching keeps us vital, enhances clarity and challenges us with questions. Often, questions from such students are the seeds of research. Whenever possible, we should find opportunities to be a mentor.

As part of maintaining an academic perspective on practice, it is also helpful for each physician to not only be a mentor, but also to find a mentor. Such a person may be located at a great distance; perhaps at the institution where his/her residency was completed; and contact may be infrequent. However, it is worth the effort it takes to maintain relationships with former teachers and role models, to visit them occasionally (preferably at their offices or homes), or at least share a meal at a meeting, and to call a valued teacher with questions and ideas. This author has never encountered a physician who considers such contacts from a colleague or former student anything other than a privilege and pleasure.

Summary

The academic practice of medicine does not end after residency, nor does it depend upon employment in an academic institution or affiliate. Academic practice is a state of mind and a mode of living. It is a commitment to intellectual vitality, and to recognizing, but never accepting, the limits of our knowledge. It is a call to keep asking questions and to pursue answers methodically; and it is a commitment for each of us to leave our field of medicine better than we found it.

References

1. Ware, M. Peer review: benefits, perceptions and alternatives. London, England: Publishing Research Consortium. 2008; pp. 1–20.
2. Mark Ware Consulting. Publishing Research Consortium Peer review survey 2015. London, England: Publishing Research Consortium 2016; pp. 1–58. https://www.elsevier.com/__data/assets/pdf_file/0007/655756/PRC-peer-review-survey-report-Final-2016-05-19.pdf. Accessed November 9, 2018.

Reprinted with modifications by permission of SAGE Publications from:

Sataloff RT. The Academic Practice of Otolaryngology: Philosophical and Practical Perspectives. *Annals of Otol Rhinol Laryngol* 2006;115(6):403–7.

4. Resident duty hours: Concerns and consequences

Physician educators have pondered optimal training paradigms for centuries. In recent years, the topic has received a great deal of attention in the United States and elsewhere. Much of the deliberation has been focused on concerns about patient safety. This emphasis is neither new nor simple. For example, the American College of Surgeons (ACS) has emphasized patient safety since its inception in 1913 and has focused its efforts primarily on patient safety throughout the first decades of the 21st century.

Resident fatigue has received wide attention as a potential threat to patient safety, and this issue has resonated particularly strongly with the general public and with legislators. The issue is complex. On the one hand, most of us who have survived surgical internship are well aware of the possibility that we might not perform at our best when we are excessively fatigued, and it seems reasonable to suspect that extreme fatigue may lead to impaired judgment and increased propensity toward medical errors. On the other hand, extensive, hands-on patient experience and continuity of care seem essential for optimal training.

In order to address concerns about excessive work-hour requirements, New York was the first state to enact duty-hour restrictions.[1] This action was followed by a report from the Institute of Medicine (IOM) of the National Academies that has had major impact on resident training.[2] In 2003, the Accreditation Council for Graduate

Medical Education (ACGME) enacted duty-hour restrictions that included a maximum work week of 80 hours. It was believed that the 80-hour work week would result in improved surgical outcomes and patient safety. Unfortunately, so far data have not demonstrated this result. The fact that no evidence-based data show that duty-hour restrictions produce better outcomes has led to ongoing reconsideration of the policy, and predictable controversy.

Among many other possibilities, some educators feel that the benefits of reduced fatigue have been offset by problems related to continuity of care and patient 'hand-off' errors. Others feel diminished clinical experience has caused problems and still more feel that the duty hours have not been reduced enough. Although we clearly need prospective, carefully designed studies on which to base future judgments regarding resident training, we are fortunate to be in a position to review the outcomes of reduced work hours in Europe and the United Kingdom.

The European Working Time Directive (EWTD) restricted duty hours more than two decades ago (October 1, 1998) and has been widely considered a failure.[3,4] The consensus is that the reduced work week (58 hours in 2004, phased to 48 hours in 2009, with 11 continuous hours of rest in each 24-hour period) has produced inadequately trained residents with insufficient experience and an unacceptably low number of surgical cases performed. The inadequate experience and insufficient emphasis on the whole patient appear to have resulted in decreased patient safety, rather than patient protection.[5]

The ACS addressed duty-hour concerns on March 4, 2008, in a presentation to the Institute of Medicine.[6] In the ACS report, in addition to patient safety and training quality, numerous other issues were discussed, including the costs involved in replacing residents (whose work hours are restricted) with other healthcare providers, in order to maintain the current level of care. Summarizing calculations in the ACS report by H. Hunt Batjer, M.D., F.A.C.S., of Northwestern University, who calculated the costs to one institution associated with a work-hour reduction to 56 hours per week (which has been discussed), it would cost about $15 million to replace lost resident/fellow hours with new residents, or about $60 million to replace them with other healthcare providers. Similar costs can be expected at other training institutions, with the impact expected to exceed $1 billion.

Replacing the lost hours with additional residents and fellows might prove impossible for a variety of reasons; and even if it were possible, it would dilute the individual resident training experience even further than it is diminished already by the work-hour restrictions. Nevertheless, the ACS recommended that the restrictive cap on federal funding of resident positions be removed in order to permit an increase in residency training positions, as an option for addressing patient care requirements.

The ACS also recommended effective team-training initiatives; the integration of advanced information technology and simulation into surgical training and healthcare delivery; exemption of the chief surgical resident from duty-hour restrictions 'to allow a more realistic transition to a postgraduate career and to acquire the knowledge and skills for practice'; and a fully funded, multi-institutional study to determine optimal duty hours. Discipline-specific outcome measures were recommended, as well.

In December 2008, the IOM issued a new document: Resident Duty Hours: Enhancing Sleep, Supervision, and Safety.[7] Medical schools and other educational institutions worked to understand the implications of that document and to implement of its recommendations. It contains some changes from the 2003 ACGME document. The ACGME established a maximum resident work time of 80 hours per week averaged over 4 weeks and limited the longest consecutive work period to 30 hours. The IOM's Committee on Optimizing Graduate Medical Trainee (Resident) Hours and Work Schedule to Improve Patient Safety reevaluated these guidelines at the request of Congress (2007) and recommended adjustments to the 2003 work rules.

So far, further reductions in the 80-hour averaged work week have not been recommended. However, other changes have, most recently in 2017.[8] Moonlighting and other employment must be counted toward the 80-hour maximum weekly hour limit, as well as at-home call. Residents must have scheduled a minimum of one day free of duty every week (when averaged over four weeks). At-home call cannot be assigned on these free days. The maximum shift length for PGY-1 residents of 16 hours with no protected sleep period has been eliminated. PGY-1 residents are restricted from moonlighting. The maximum for PGY-2 residents and above may be scheduled to a maximum of 24 hours, with no additional clinical responsibilities after 24 hours of continuous in-house duty, although they may remain on-site for an additional four hours for patient safety issues such as patient care transition or education. Residents must not be scheduled for more than six consecutive night shifts. PGY-2 residents and above must be scheduled for in-house call no more frequently than every-third night (when averaged over a four-week period). Time spent in the hospital and on at-home call must count towards the 80-hour maximum weekly hour limit. The frequency of at-home call is not subject to the every-third-night limitation, but it must satisfy the requirement for one-day-in-seven free of duty, when averaged over four weeks. Residents' minimum time off between clinical or educational periods is eight hours. Residents must have at least 14 hours free of duty after 24 hours of in-house duty. There is no longer a 6-night limit on the frequency of in-hospital night float duty. Strategic napping, especially after 16 hours of continuous duty and between the hours of 10:00pm and 8:00am, is suggested strongly. In unusual circumstances, residents, on their own initiative, may remain beyond their scheduled period of duty to continue to provide care to a single patient. Justifications for such extensions of duty are limited to reasons of required continuity of care for a severely ill or unstable patient, academic importance of the events transpiring, or humanistic attention to the needs of a patient or family. Reading, studying and academic preparation away from the hospital are not counted as duty hours. Unfortunately, there still is no convincing evidence that these policies have improved patient safety, and concerns persist about their adverse effects on resident education.

While not on enforcement of the various regulations regarding resident duty hours, a few issues are worthy of thought. The ACGME is enforcing the duty hours through careful monitoring, direct contact with trainees, site visits, and the standard residency approval processes.

There have been discussions by some legislators about enacting laws that would criminalize violations. There is already a law in New Jersey, enacted in August 2003, that affects the definition of criminal homicide by vehicle in that state.[9] This law presumes impairment if a driver has been awake for 24 consecutive hours or more and is involved in a motor vehicle accident resulting in a fatality. The implications for a resident involved in such a situation are obvious, as well as those for an institution that required, or permitted, a resident to work for a 24-hour period. It seems likely that we will encounter other legislative efforts (possibly at a federal level) to address the public's growing (if not fully informed) concern over duty hours.

It also seems worthwhile to consider other potential consequences of the concern over this issue. These are my speculation and have not been discussed widely to the best of my knowledge, but I believe they are worth considering. First, airline safety protocols have been discussed frequently as models for medical safety protocols. Carrying the analogy further, it seems worth noting that we (post-residency physicians) are the captains of the ship. If the government joins our regulatory agencies in controlling work hours of trainees in the name of patient safety, it might be only a matter of time before someone considers controlling the work hours of physicians who are ultimately responsible for those trainees and their patient care. I would anticipate that we will be confronted with this perplexing challenge eventually, and it might be worthwhile for us to consider it and plan for it in advance.

Second, while we are altering resident training protocols, especially if we consider reducing work hours further (65-hour and 56-hour work weeks have been mentioned), we will need to look at the implications for the relationship between physicians and other allied healthcare professionals. In the Commonwealth of Pennsylvania, for example, numerous bills have been introduced into the legislature to expand the scope of practice of non-physician allied healthcare personnel. Many have passed.

Nurse anesthetists currently are lobbying strongly for the ability to deliver anesthesia without physician supervision. Several years ago, nurse practitioners in Pennsylvania tried to introduce a bill (it did not make it to the floor) expanding their scope of practice to include unsupervised surgery (tonsillectomy and appendectomy were to be included). Their argument was that they were the only healthcare providers in underserved areas of rural Pennsylvania and should be able to perform these procedures that used to be within the scope of the traditional family physician. Their initial effort to gain these practice privileges was not successful. However, if resident work hours were to be reduced further and surgical residents were trained in a 65- or 56-hour work environment, over 5 or 10 years the difference between a physician-surgeon and a nurse practitioner with additional surgical training would narrow substantially. This, coupled with the emphasis on less-expensive providers, might change substantially the rationale for the current scope of practice determinations. In my opinion, it also would have frightening implications for patient safety.

The resident duty-hour issue is important not only for those of us involved with resident education, but moreover for anyone who practices medicine or who might require medical care as a patient sometime in the future. That means that all of us need not only to stay familiar with current developments, but also to look into the future for the potential long-term implications. Our ability to continue practicing medicine of the highest quality and our ability to offer our patients safe, excellent care is at stake; and it might be in jeopardy.

References

1. Asch DA, Parker RM. The Libby Zion case. One step forward or two steps backward? *N Engl J Med* 1988;318(12):771–5.
2. Kohn LT, Corrigan JM, Donaldson MS, eds. Committee on Quality of Health Care in America, Institute of Medicine. To Err is Human: Building a Safer Health System. Washington, DC: The National Academies Press; 2000.
3. Benes V. The European Working Time Directive and the effects on training of surgical specialists (doctors in training): A position paper of the surgical disciplines of the countries of the EU. *Acta Neurochir* (Wien) 2006;148(11):1227–33.
4. Marron C, Shah J, Mole D, Slade D. ASIT opinion on the European Working Time Directive (EWTD). The Association of Surgeons in Training at the Royal College of Surgeons of England. London, UK, May 2006.
5. William E.G. Thomas, MS, FRCS, Chairman of Education for the Royal College of Surgeons of England. Personal communication with Josef E. Fischer

(1/22/08). [As cited in Position of the American College of Surgeons on Restrictions on Resident Work Hours. *Bull Am Coll Surg* 2009;94(1):11–18].
6. American College of Surgeons Task Force on the Resident 80-hour Work Week. Position of the American College of Surgeons on Restrictions on Resident Work Hours. *Bull Am Coll Surg* 2009;94(1):11–8.
7. Ulmer C, Miller Wolman D, Johns MME, eds. Committee on Optimizing Graduate Medical Trainee (Resident) Hours and Work Schedule to Improve Patient Safety, National Research Council. Resident Duty Hours: Enhancing Sleep, Supervision, and Safety. Washington, DC: The National Academies Press; 2008.
8. Summary of Changes to ACGME Common Program Requirements Section VI. Accreditation Council for Graduate Medical Education 2018. http://www.acgme.org/What-We-Do/Accreditation/Common-Program-Requirements/Summary-of-Proposed-Changes-to-ACGME-Common-Program-Requirements-Section-VI. [Accessed July 2018].
9. New Jersey Senate Bill No. 1644. https://legiscan.com/NJ/text/S1644/id/1719394/New_Jersey-2018-S1644-Introduced.html. [Accessed August 20, 2018].

Reprinted with modifications by permission of Vendome Group from:
 Sataloff RT. Resident duty hours: Concerns and consequences. *ENT J* 2009;88(3):812–6.

5. Consistency of medical student education: Otolaryngology as a model for medical student subspecialty training

Educating medical students is one of the most important responsibilities and privileges of any physician affiliated with a medical school. Offering an excellent, diverse, exciting educational experience for medical students is important for many reasons. Such educational adventures have inspired many medical students to enter general practice specialties; and a continuing supply of excellent residency applicants requires a continuing supply of medical students who are excited by what they have learned and seen during rotations.

Attention to educational excellence is essential not only in large, core fields such as internal medicine and surgery, but also in smaller specialties such as otolaryngology, for example. Outstanding medical student experience will continue to inspire the 'top of the class' to seek training in otolaryngology; but such education is critical for other students who pursue other disciplines, as well. Not only is it important for us to teach them the breadth and diversity of Otolaryngology-Head & Neck Surgery so that they understand what otolaryngologists do and which patients should be referred for otolaryngologic consultation, but it is also critical for us to equip them with a core body of knowledge. Medical students who enter other specialties will treat many people with head and neck complaints ranging from colds, to hearing loss, to dizziness, to facial paralysis, to many other common afflictions. We are obligated to teach medical students enough to understand the complexities of our field, the basic management of otolaryngologic disorders and, most importantly, how to recognize problems that exceed their expertise so that they can educate themselves further and/or make appropriate and timely referrals.

In many medical schools, we have three weeks or less of medical student contact to achieve these goals, sometimes augmented by a few clinical correlation lectures and a couple of hours of physical examination training ('gag lab') during the first year or two of medical school.

As if this challenge weren't daunting enough, otolaryngology chairs and program directors are commonly faced with another logistic, academic and political situation that often compounds the difficulty of assuring good education. In many medical schools, clinical education is conducted at multiple affiliate sites.

In some cities, the medical student (and resident) experience at affiliate hospitals may equal or even exceed that at the university hospital (although often this is not the case), but there are invariably differences among various training sites. This can make it difficult not only to ensure reasonably comparable exposure to otolaryngologic diagnosis and surgery, but also to ensure comparable acquisition of core knowledge about otolaryngology at all sites.

Ideally, all affiliate sites are within easy commuting distance of the home institution, and students can spend an academic day or half-day at the university listening to lectures, taking advantage of research and publication opportunities, comparing experience at the different sites (among themselves and with faculty), and recognizing and compensating for any training gaps. However, at many medical schools, some rotation sites are too far distant to permit this approach. For example, although Drexel University College of Medicine is based in Philadelphia, we have academic campuses two hours away in northern New Jersey, and 300 miles away in Pittsburgh and 3,000 miles away in California. Those centers have good case volume and are staffed by excellent otolaryngologists, or they would not be affiliate training sites; but the availability and consistency of didactic training vary.

Perhaps the most obvious solution to the problem would be videoconference lectures and rounds. While these sound like a good idea and should be encouraged, they present practical difficulties because of the different schedules and commitments at each site, as well as time zone differences. They also may generate costs related to videoconferencing equipment and personnel (depending on the policies of each institution) for which funds usually have not been budgeted. This arrangement also can inspire disagreement about whether such funding should be provided by the hospital, the medical school, the department, or some other source. Once commitments have been made and funds spent, there also may be repercussions if a faculty member has to cancel a lecture at the last minute.

While interactive videoconferencing is an excellent educational tool, we also have found online training to be practical. While the technology for this approach has been available for many years, it has not been adopted in otolaryngology as widely as might be desirable. This author suggests that this approach is worthy of consideration and expansion within our curricula.

In many institutions, residents and faculty give the same lectures to medical students every month. This means leaving the office or operating room. Most lectures are good, but the lectures given by the chief resident one year are always somewhat different from the lectures on the same topic given by previous or subsequent chief residents; and it is impossible for the content of every lecture to be reviewed in detail by faculty unless all of the lectures are given by faculty. This is problematic even with single-site education. It also is questionable whether it is the best possible use of resident and faculty time, or the most useful educational process for the students.

In Philadelphia, we have changed the paradigm. Each medical student is required to listen to 12 online lectures and take a written examination on their content. These lectures were prepared by faculty and produced professionally. They can be taken at the convenience of the student, at times even before his/her otolaryngology rotation begins, if the student is sufficiently motivated. If there were a generally accepted, short, practical otolaryngology text designed to permit the study of otolaryngology during a two-to- three-week rotation, it might provide an acceptable alternative. However, most of the current texts provide more information than students can absorb without guidance. In addition, many current students find online education convenient, and they are comfortable with it. Requiring that this core knowledge be obtained through standardized online lectures provides a way of equalizing acquisition of core knowledge among the sites. Moreover, it allows faculty and residents to spend their time with the students discussing cases, pursuing problem-based learning, and interacting in ways that seem more meaningful than didactic lectures transmitting knowledge that can be learned equally well before students and faculty meet face-to-face.

Resources such as the online lectures are becoming more widely available. Our lectures were developed for the Graduate Education Foundation (GEF), a nonprofit organization accredited by the Accreditation Council for Continuing Medical Education. The otolaryngology lectures are 12 of approximately 130 lectures developed as CME offerings for family practitioners. The GEF (in which I have no commercial interest other than being a contributing author and unpaid advisor) made these 130 lectures available for educational institutions at little cost, but the organization ceased to exist and all video lectures are now available only through their authors.

While these core lectures should not be considered a comprehensive education in otolaryngology, they do provide a start toward solving the problem of providing consistent, faculty-approved core knowledge to otolaryngology students. They also may be a useful starting point for other departments as they develop their own online materials. Such lectures are also extremely valuable for office staff, nurses, audiologists, and other interested colleagues. They have been received well by new otolaryngology residents as they enter our program, and by residents who rotate with us routinely from the departments of pulmonary medicine, family medicine, and ambulatory medicine.

It is important for each otolaryngology department to be comfortable that every medical student who completes an otolaryngology rotation has been exposed to the core body of knowledge that each chair considers essential for every practitioner of medicine.

The author has not addressed the issue of consistency between institutions, or the advisability of adopting a national curriculum and agreeing on what constitutes minimum core information. That challenging topic should be addressed in the future. However, standard use of faculty-approved online lectures and formal testing has proven useful to our students, residents, and faculty. Further consideration and development of this approach seem warranted.

Reprinted with modifications by permission of Vendome Group from:
Sataloff RT. Consistency of medical student education in otolaryngology. *ENT J* 2009;88(1):714–7.

6. Fellowship training in otolaryngology

Otolaryngology–Head & Neck Surgery offers one of the most sought-after residencies in medicine. Most otolaryngology residencies are excellent and essentially, all provide comprehensive training that prepares graduates to provide superb clinical care. Despite the high quality of residency training, fellowship training has become increasingly popular. In some subspecialties (neurotology, for example), additional clinical training is required to develop competence in advanced procedures. However, in other specialties (such as head and neck surgery), graduates of many programs already have substantial skill and experience when they complete their residencies. It is interesting to speculate about the factors driving young otolaryngologists to pursue additional training and the implications of this pattern for the future of otolaryngology and possibly, other disciplines.

For better or worse, young otolaryngologists are influenced by those of us who serve as mentors. Many otolaryngology residency programs are staffed by academic otolaryngologists who are subspecialists. We serve as role models. Many of us encourage our trainees to pursue additional fellowship training, and it is widely regarded as an almost-necessary prerequisite to a career in academic otolaryngology. Most educators encourage trainees to consider careers in academic medicine in the hope that they will pass on the training we have provided for them and advance the field over the course of their careers. Academic medicine is attractive to many young otolaryngologists not only for intellectual reasons, but also because the burdens of running a private practice business have increased in recent years and the financial disparity between private practice and academic practice has narrowed. Hence, a desire to be competitive for an academic position undoubtedly drives many residents' decisions to pursue fellowship training. There are approximately 300 trainees finishing annually. Approximately 40% pursue additional training.

The need for additional knowledge is another important factor for many, of course. Most residencies do not provide sufficient hands-on experience in intracranial surgery to permit a graduate to practice neurotology without fellowship training. In head and neck oncologic surgery, even though many residencies provide extensive experience, fellowship training offers additional research opportunities and additional experience in complex head and neck procedures, such as free-flap surgery, for those who need the additional exposure. Additional training is also helpful after many residency experiences in fields such as facial plastic, reconstructive and cosmetic surgery, laryngology, rhinology and pediatric otolaryngology.

A review of fellowship programs available to otolaryngologists highlights the scope of our field. Fellowships are available currently in allergy and immunology, cosmetic surgery, facial plastic and reconstructive surgery, head and neck oncology, laryngology/voice, otology, neurotology, and skull base surgery, pediatric otolaryngology, rhinology and sleep medicine. In addition, some otolaryngology graduates pursue a second residency in plastic and reconstructive surgery.

There is a place for general otolaryngologists who graduate from residency programs and provide high quality care to communities, and there will always be need for such practitioners in community and in university environments. However, even in community private-practice settings, there is an increasing tendency to subspecialize within practices. Sometimes special interest in a subspecialty, coupled with good residency training, is sufficient to prepare practitioners to be the 'go to' person for ear problems, voice problems, head and neck cancer, or other special issues within a practice. However, even outside academic settings, there may be a benefit to pursuing an organized, efficient, and comprehensive fellowship in a physician's area of interest. Within the academic world, such fellowship trained subspecialists form the core of our educational programs. They are also the driving force behind clinical and basic subspecialty research that is advancing our field.

While there have been discussions for more than 40 years about changes in our training paradigm, it seems likely that as we continue to attract the best and brightest medical graduates to the field of otolaryngology–head and neck surgery, there will continue to be a substantial number of bright, young otolaryngologists who want to know everything there is to know about their area of subspecialty interest. These are likely to be the same physicians who will help us learn those things that we do not yet know. Hence, it seems probable that the trend toward fellowship training will continue, and that it will enhance otolaryngologic care for all patients, not only by inspiring new research and providing tertiary subspecialty care, but also by improving training in otolaryngology–head and neck surgery for all of our graduates, regardless of the career paths that they choose. Recognizing the importance of fellowship training, it would probably be wise for our specialty to review the nature and consistency of fellowship training in the various subspecialty areas. This is particularly true of those that are not approved by the American Board of Medical Specialties and eligible for training program approval by the American College of Graduate Medical Education (only neurotology, pediatric otolaryngology, plastic surgery within the head and neck, and sleep medicine have ACGME program approval available), and therefore might not be following a prescribed and relatively standardized curriculum.

We have passed the time in our history when we should be willing to tolerate great disparity among programs in the same subspecialty area. In the absence of formal certification programs, it seems timely for us to consider developing at least core curricula for each of the subspecialty areas, and possibly oversight groups to provide certificates (if not certification) to fellowship programs that comply. Such guiding bodies could be developed by the Academy, subspecialty societies, committees of all program directors, the Society of University Otolaryngologists or a combination thereof; but it is time for the sophistication and consistency of fellowship program guidance and oversight to catch up with the popularity and importance of fellowship training.

Reprinted with modifications by permission of Vendome Group from:
    Sataloff RT. Fellowship training in otolaryngology. *ENT J* 2009;88(9):1084–6.

7. Interdisciplinary opportunities for creativity in medicine

In the Hippocratic oath, we swear: 'I will keep pure and holy both my life and my art.' From time to time, it behooves us to reflect upon our lives in medicine and to assess not only whether we have remained true to our original mission, but also whether our profession still provides viable possibilities for altruistic, creative practice.

Observations at different stages of medical education reveal disturbing trends. Pre-medical students are usually enthusiastically committed to helping mankind, not only by aiding one patient at a time, but also by advancing medical science. Physicians who have been in practice for a number of years speak much more often of malpractice crises, overhead expenses, managed care, and the changing politics of medical practice.

In the past several years, more and more young, successful doctors have begun seeking alternative careers - outside of medicine. The purpose of this chapter is not to analyze the educational and cultural factors that turn so many bright-eyed, idealistic pre-meds into so many jaded, pragmatic doctors (nearly all of us have our own theories). Certainly, the demands of our profession make it hard enough for most of us to keep up with the necessities of patient care and running our practices or departments. Stimulating, novel ideas and imaginative new approaches to medical treatment are often not a part of our daily routines. Yet, many of us expected that they would be. This author believes that it is still possible and preferable to incorporate creative imagination into everyday practice. This can be accomplished with slight adjustments in philosophy and traditional practice methods. Interdisciplinary teamwork is a particularly satisfactory approach.

For hundreds of years, medical doctors have practiced alone. For some, especially in earlier times, this was done to protect their mystique and because of their insecurities. For others, isolation was a consequence of specialization. This is not a new phenomenon. Herodotus (484–424 B.C.) wrote:

The art of medicine in Egypt is thus exercised: one physician is confined to the study and management of one disease; there are of course a great number who practice this art; some attend to the disorders of the eyes, others to those of the head, some take care of the teeth, others are conversant with all diseases of the bowels; whilst many attend to the cure of maladies which are less conspicuous.

The old tradition continues today, even in most university settings and multispecialty groups. Although doctors work together under the same roof and talk together in the same conference rooms, they rarely truly think together and work together as a unit. It is even more rare for them to interact with nonphysicians in a meaningful way.

However, in the last several years, an encouraging number of new interdisciplinary teams have emerged. They are important not merely because of their advances in medical treatment, but also because of their changes in thinking, cooperation and approaches to caring for patients. Collaboration has resulted in new opportunities for creative approaches to medical problems, approaches that were not possible to adopt from the parochial posture of isolated specialists.

The team approach

The team concept in medicine is certainly not entirely new. For example, in-depth cooperation among internists and surgeons made cardiac surgery and renal transplantation possible. More recently, cooperation among radiologists and neurosurgeons has resulted in intraoperative ultrasound localization of brain lesions, invasive radiologic treatment of stenoses and aneurysms, and other major advances that have improved safety and decreased morbidity. Sports medicine has combined the skills and insights of various specialists to revolutionize the care of professional athletes. Selected spinal cord injury 'teams' have combined the talents of neurosurgeons and orthopedic surgeons, operating on the same patient at the same time, along with the skills of physiatrists, physical therapists, psychologists, speech-language pathologists, and others. Such collaboration results in a dialogue and subtle refinements of ideas that are rare for the physician working alone.

Learning to work together, being open to different ideas and approaches, and being prepared to make time to talk with a colleague are among the most important requirements of the interdisciplinary team. The physicians must replace egotistical prerogatives with genuine, open curiosity. This posture allows a fresh approach to old problems, armed with new perspectives and divested of the boundaries of traditional specialties and their limitations.

This author has been fortunate enough to be involved with two such interdisciplinary teams throughout his career. They keep the practice of medicine exciting and vital. The newest frontier in otology is the ear–brain interface, the skull base. It was an unexplored boundary full of vital structures that represented the limit of otolaryngology, coming from below, and the boundary of neurosurgery, coming from above. Unraveling the mysteries of the 'no-man's land' of the skull base has become possible only in the last four decades because of the interdisciplinary specialty of neurotology. This subspecialty had its beginnings in Los Angeles, in the early 1960s, for the treatment of acoustic neuromas and glomus tumors. It led to the development of the cochlear implant, surgical cures for vertigo, and other advances. More recently, it also has led to major new developments in the treatment of previously 'unresectable' malignancies of the temporal bone, and to expanded approaches to all areas of the skull base involving other specialists, such as rhinologists.

Our team includes not only a neurotologist (the author) and neurosurgeon, but also an ophthalmologist, internist, general surgeon, anesthesiologist, psychiatrist, nurse, rehabilitation specialist, and others attuned to the special problems of these patients and their prolonged surgeries. Consequently, since 1980, we have been able to develop new techniques with which to resect areas that have not been resected before, to manage anesthesia safely for more than 30 hours when necessary, and to return patients to their homes, self-sufficient and in reasonably good condition. Moreover, every time we do such a case, we find new ways to do it better. Occasionally, we find techniques to do more things that we thought were not possible. Such interactions help to keep the joy in medical practice.

Arts medicine

Not all creative teamwork has to involve 30-hour operations and critically ill patients. The interdisciplinary specialty of arts medicine has also evolved remarkably since its introduction in the 1980s. There is already an International Arts Medicine Association, and there are arts medicine clinics and conferences in several states. This field is exciting for a variety of reasons. First, performers and artists place extreme demands on their bodies and do not have the usual tolerance for incomplete cures.

An injured finger that returns to 98% normal function might be adequate even for a microsurgeon, but not for a premier pianist. That extra 2% separates the famous artist from the artist who has not quite reached the 'top'.

The author has been involved extensively with the treatment of singers and other professional voice users since the late 1970s. Learning how to recognize, define and treat subtleties of voice pathology that are not even mentioned in many residency programs, has been a daily challenge and joy. Much of the fun and many of the ideas have come from close collaboration with speech-language pathologists, singing teachers, acting voice teachers, voice scientists, and other colleagues, all of whom provide insights useful in clinical practice. Second, arts medicine provides physicians with an opportunity to work closely with professionals in the arts and humanities. Not all 'interdisciplinary opportunities' need to be among medical disciplines.

Arts and medicine are inherently similar in many ways. However, through our educational process, physicians too often lose sight of the importance of arts and humanities in our practices. There is a movement in medical education to correct this problem and arts medicine offers the clinician a chance to work and think with colleagues in related fields, with artists and performers, and to find new solutions to complex problems. It also may afford the inspiration and opportunity to study one of the arts.

As A.M. Harvey wrote in his book *The Principles and Practice of Medicine*, 'The principal complaint which patients make about modern scientific medicine is the failure of physicians to communicate with them adequately'. Tolstoy observed that, 'Art is the human activity having for its purpose the transmission to others of the highest and best feelings to which men have risen'. In our quest to master the science and art of healing, we can learn much from our colleagues in the arts and humanities that will enhance our insight, sensitivity and ability to empathize.

True interdisciplinary study provides endless opportunity for the enrichment of the practice of medicine with creative insights. Whether we work with tertiary care surgeons to resect the 'unresectable', or with poets to find new ways to hear and talk with our distraught patients, medicine remains a viable option for the imaginative, creative physician who still wants the same exciting challenges and opportunities he or she wanted as a sophomore in college. We need only refuse to accept anything less.

Reprinted with modifications by permission of Vendome Group from:

Sataloff RT. Interdisciplinary opportunities for creativity in medicine. *ENT J* 1998;77(7):530–533.

8. Physicians studying voice and the arts

Much has been said about the necessity for interdisciplinary education. Speech-language pathologists, acting teachers and singing teachers clearly need to study anatomy, physiology, and basic health maintenance of the voice. Singing teachers need to learn about the speaking voice. Speech-language pathologists benefit from singing study, voice scientists need to understand clinical problems and priorities, and so forth. At the most practical level, the reasons why a laryngologist should study voice are obvious. Through singing lessons, speech lessons, and personal performance experience, we acquire terminology, experience, and understanding that cannot be achieved in other ways; this makes us better doctors. Without such training, the laryngologist can compensate to some degree by reading and study, but he or she never acquires quite the same expertise or patient rapport as the physician, who also has experienced the discipline of musical development and the ecstasy and terror of public performance.

However, there may be even more compelling reasons for physicians to study the arts in general. Many of the most rewarding joys of subspecializing in voice or other areas of arts-medicine come from the interdisciplinary opportunities for creativity and the philosophical influence of our colleagues in the humanities. It is wise and rewarding for physicians to recognize the importance of the study of arts in making us not only better doctors, but also better people.

A modern poet has characterized the personality of art and the personality of science as: 'Art is I: Science is We'.[1]

Since its earliest days, medicine has concerned itself with refining its understanding of the truths of science and art and applying their universal wisdom to the care of people. This implies an obligation for the physician to understand more about life than just the particulars of body function with which our science is concerned. We must expand our parochial vision into a broad understanding of humanity. One of the most obvious and accessible avenues to such philosophical breadth is the combination of medical studies with the study of the arts.

'Only though art can we get outside ourselves and know another's view of the universe which is not the same as ours and see landscapes which would otherwise have remained unknown to us like the landscapes of the moon. Thanks to art, instead of seeing a single world, our own, we see it multiply until we have before us as many worlds as there are original artists'.[2] Understanding the arts of poetry, music, painting and other forms of deep expression helps sophisticate our art of understanding.

David, da Vinci, Shakespeare, Bach, and others of their stature have remained vital because of the depth and universality of their visions of life. Understanding their messages enriches our entire being and gives new light to our own vision. Moreover, the process of learning to understand their wisdom teaches us how to perceive another's view - the art of understanding. As physicians, we must believe that there are as many 'original artists' as there are people in the world and it is the art of our profession to see what they see and to care for them accordingly.

'The principal complaint which patients make about 'modern science medicine' is the failure of physicians to communicate with them adequately', wrote Osler.[3] What patients are trying to tell us is not that they want more information, but that they want more humanity.

'Art is the human activity having for its purpose the transmission to others of the highest and best feelings to which men have risen'.[4] This fundamental caring is what we fail too often to communicate. This is especially curious, since it is what draws so many of us to medicine and makes it so much more fulfilling for us than the laboratory sciences. If we fail to communicate our feelings with our patients or to understand the feelings that they communicate to us, then we fail as physicians. Studying the arts can be invaluable in teaching us to communicate and to understand not only what our patients are saying, but also what they are not saying.

In addition to more abstract wisdom, study of the arts reveals a rather reassuring similarity of methods among the arts and sciences, as well as a similarity of goals.

> He who would do good to another must do it in minute particulars:
> General Good is the plea of the scoundrel, hypocrite and flatterer,
> For art and science cannot exist but in minutely organized particulars.[5]

Both science and art seek universal truths; both seek the 'I' and the 'We' and both recognize that the substance of great truths is smaller truths. Only their perspectives differ. Moreover, mastery of these differences may well be the substance of the genius that allows a few people occasionally to see that which has been before all of us all of the time but has been missed.

We swear in the Hippocratic Oath: 'I will keep pure and holy both my life and my art'. In our quest to master the science of art and healing, we will do well to pay attention to the nature of the lives and world with which we live and especially to art, the science of the study of that nature. 'It is art that makes life, makes interest, makes importance, for our consideration and application of these things, and I know no substitute whatever for the force and the beauty of its process'.[6] As Hippocrates observed, 'Where there is love of man, there is also love of the art'.[4] If we are to master the art of medicine, study of the arts may provide invaluable help, for to have the love is not enough. We must learn to understand it and to communicate it to our patients so that they feel it. This is where our science fails; and without this art, we are about as comforting as a well-programmed computer, and not nearly so efficient.

It is somewhat comforting, and somewhat humbling, to consider one final truth:

> All nature is but art unknown to thee,
> All chance direction which thou canst not see;
> All discord, harmony not understood;
> All partial evil, universal good;
> And spite of pride, in erring reason's spite,
> One truth is clear, Whatever is, is right.[8]

References

1. Bernard C. Art is I: Science is We. *Bull NYAcad Med IV*. 1928;1V:997.
2. Proust M. O'Brien J, ed. *The Maxims of Marcel Proust*. New York, New York: Columbia University Press; 1948:235.
3. Harvey AM, Johns RJ, Owens AH, Ross RS. *The Principles and Practice of Medicine*, 18th ed. New York, New York: Appleton-Century-Crofts, 1972:2.
4. Tolstoy L. *What Is Art?* 1898:chap 8.
5. Blake W. *Jerusalem*. Chapter 3, Sec. 55.
6. James H. *Letter to H.G. Wells*, July 10, 1915.
7. Pope A. *An essay on man*. Epistle 1:289.
8. Hippocrates. *Precepts*. Chapter 1.

Reprinted with modifications by permission of Plural Publishing, Inc. from:
Sataloff RT. Physicians studying voice and the arts. In: Sataloff RT. *Professional Voice: The Science and Art of Clinical Care*, 4th ed. San Diego, California: Plural

Publishing, Inc., 2017: pp. 1851–2; and, reprinted with modifications by permission of Vendome Group from:

Sataloff RT. Physicians: The importance of studying the arts. *ENT J* 2004; 83(4):212.

9. Arts medicine: An interdisciplinary paradigm

Health hazards in the arts have been recognized at least since 1713 when Bernardino Ramazzini published *Diseases of Tradesmen*,[1] and there have been sporadic publications on various related subjects over the past three centuries.[2] However, the concepts of arts medicine have evolved into a medical specialty, primarily since the late 1970s and early 1980s. Many of the best-known advances in the field focus on the problems of performing artists.[3-5] But equally important and dramatic advances also have occurred in the visual arts. Arts medicine has exerted an impact not only through medical improvements, but also through heightened awareness of health hazards among artists and improving artistic training and practice. Much important new information has been amassed. Medicine, the arts, and related disciplines are now faced with the challenge of disseminating information, educating practitioners in all fields, and creating an environment in which the arts can be practiced with the fewest possible adverse health consequences.

A great many musicians have health problems. Questionnaires were sent to 4,025 professional musicians with affiliate orchestras of the International Conference of Symphony and Opera Musicians (ICSOM), of which 2,212 questionnaires were returned.[6] Of the musicians responding, 82% reported medical problems and 76% had a medical problem that adversely affected performance. Many of these musicians had problems caused or aggravated by musical performance. Yet, until the past few decades, this was not widely known, and musicians were afraid to admit their difficulties for fear of losing work. Moreover, those who did seek medical attention usually were disappointed with the evaluation and results.

When world-class pianist Gary Graffman developed difficulty controlling his right hand, he persevered until he found a physician who was willing to look at the possibility that his problem was caused by playing the piano. Together, they began to understand his overuse syndrome. When Graffman made his difficulties known to the general public and Leon Fleischer followed suit, thousands of musicians discovered they were not alone and began to seek help. Gradually, the medical profession has learned to provide the care musicians need. Moreover, farsighted music schools are beginning to incorporate scientifically based practice techniques in their curricula.

For physicians, arts medicine and sports medicine pose special interests, challenges and problems. Traditional medical training has not provided the background necessary to address them well. Consequently, the development of these fields has required understanding and interaction among physicians, performers or athletes, and members of other disciplines. Such cooperation and interaction have taken so long to develop largely because of language barriers. For example, when a singer complains of a 'thready midrange', most doctors do not know what he or she is talking about. To the traditional physician, if such a singer looks healthy and has vocal folds that appear normal on mirror examination, he or she is deemed normal by the physician.

Medicine, in general, enjoys a broad range of physical condition that is considered 'normal'. The biggest difference we encounter in arts and sports medicine is the performer or athlete's sophisticated self-analysis and narrow definition of normal. In general, doctors are not trained to recognize and work with the last few percent of optimal physical performance. The arts medicine specialist is trained to discern subtle differences in the supranormal to near perfect range, in which the professional performer's body must operate.

To really understand performers, physicians must either be performers themselves, or work closely with performers, teachers, coaches, trainers, and specific paramedical professionals. In voice, for example, this means a laryngologist works with a singing teacher, voice coach, voice trainer, voice scientist, speech-language pathologist, and often other professionals. In other fields, the specialists vary, but the principles remain the same.

Caring for patients who are performers, such as professional singers and actors, is not only fun but also extremely educational for physicians. By challenging us to refine our definition of 'normal', they require us to observe more acutely, measure function and outcomes more accurately, and scrutinize our therapeutic responses more critically. These challenges, combined with what we learn through collaborating with professionals in other disciplines, make us better doctors, and this 'outside the box' approach is continuing to improve the standard of care for all of our patients, not only the performing artists who have inspired us.

References

1. Goodman H, ed. Bernardino Ramazzini: *Diseases of Tradesmen*. New York, New York: Medical Lay Press, 1933.
2. Harman SE. The evolution of performing arts medicine. In: Sataloff RT, Brandfonbrener AG, Lederman RJ, eds. *Textbook of Performing Arts Medicine* New York, New York: Raven Press, 1991:7–18.
3. Sataloff RT, Brandfonbrener AG, Lederman RJ, eds. *Textbook of Performing Arts Medicine*. New York, New York: Raven Press, 1991.
4. Sataloff RT, Brandfonbrener AG, Lederman RJ, eds. *Performing Arts Medicine*, 2nd ed. San Diego, California: Singular Publishing Group, 1998.
5. Sataloff RT, Brandfonbrener AG, Lederman RJ, eds. *Performing Arts Medicine*, 3rd ed. Narberth, Pennsylvania: Science and Medicine; 2010.
6. Fishbein M, Middlestadt SE, Ottati V, et al. Medical Problems Among ICSOM Musicians: Overview of a National Survey. *Medical Problems in the Performing Arts*. 1988;3:1–8.

Reprinted with modifications by permission of Vendome Group from:
 Sataloff RT. Arts medicine: An interdisciplinary paradigm. *ENT J* 2005;84(8):462.

10. Education in laryngology: Rising to old challenges

Education in Laryngology has been a subject of interest ever since Louis Elsberg's address to the first meeting of the American Laryngological Association in 1879. Remarkable scientific, technological, and clinical advances in recent decades have elevated the standard of laryngological care. It is essential for training programs to promulgate these important advances through well-planned, comprehensive curricula. Such training also should foster an appreciation for the kinds of creative thought, interdisciplinary collaboration, and imaginative clinical practice that have been responsible for many of the recent dramatic advances in the field of laryngology.

Introduction and historical perspective

As the field of laryngology continues to evolve, it seems appropriate to ask whether education in laryngology and voice has kept pace with the remarkable clinical and technological advances of the last few decades. Throughout the history of otolaryngology, considerable time and thought have been devoted to educational issues. The founders of the American Laryngological Association (ALA) were deeply concerned with training in laryngology. This was the subject of Louis Elsberg's Presidential Address at the first meeting of the ALA on June 10, 1879, in New York.[1] Elsberg had begun teaching laryngology in 1861, and he established the first training clinic affiliated with any institution, in 1863, at the University of the City of New York. By 1879, when the ALA was formed, Elsberg reported that there were 25 laryngology teachers in American medical schools. Elsberg's extraordinary address (57 published pages) provides a fascinating review of the history of laryngology and culminates with a section entitled 'Laryngological Instruction'. Elsberg reviewed the mission of laryngology, and of the ALA in particular, as being not only to develop greater knowledge and skills, but also to disseminate them and raise the standard of care and education. Elsberg's address to the second meeting of the ALA was delivered by Jacob Solis-Cohen, in Elsberg's absence.[2] Elsberg dedicated that entire address to specific training issues, including requirements for basic science, and clinical knowledge that should be acquired before physicians in training are permitted to care for patients. He was an advocate for both undergraduate and graduate education in laryngology and even proposed instruction in comparative laryngology to enhance the understanding of the human larynx through the study of other species. In his presidential address before the fourth meeting of the ALA, Frederick Knight emphasized the same concerns. He observed, 'It will be a great gain when every physician feels he must own a laryngoscope. A more important point for us arises, how we can make him use it intelligently; how all men who graduate from our medical schools shall be given a little available knowledge of laryngology during their precious time of pupilage.'[3] Knight stressed the importance of both didactic education and laboratory and clinical training. He also recognized the expense of medical training and called for endowment of medical schools to support education, an uncommon notion in his day. In addition, Knight offered specific recommendations for the teaching of laryngology within the medical school curriculum, even courageously calling for an extension of the duration of medical study. In Birmingham, England, in 1890, John St Swithin Wilders addressed the section of laryngology and rhinology of the British Medical Association in 'On the teaching of Laryngology'.[4] He, too, emphasized the importance of educating all physicians in the fundamentals of laryngology and use of the laryngoscope, and raised concerns about specialty hospitals, especially those that were not used by medical students in their education. He stressed the importance of laryngological education within general hospitals 'which profess to educate students' and even raised an extremely controversial call 'that no more special hospitals will be founded.'[4]

Concerns about laryngology and its place in medical education were highlighted again in Henry L. Swain's Presidential Address to the 23rd meeting of the ALA, in which he called for specific time within the medical school curriculum for courses in our field.[5] Since that time, training issues have been addressed sporadically. For example, in 1906, Knight[6] reviewed the state of training in laryngology, highlighting the proliferation of instrumentation. Reflecting back on Elsberg's day, Knight noted that the meager armamentarium offered in the olden time is in striking contrast with the vast collection of apparatus now at our command. 'It is not certain that the enormous multiplication of instruments in recent years brings marked advantage'.[6] It would be interesting to hear his perspective if he were alive today amid technological developments that make his own armamentarium look meager indeed.

Thomas J. Harris[7] addressed the complex issues of postgraduate training in laryngology in an insightful paper read before the ALA in 1913. Residency programs as we know them had not yet been developed. Harris emphasized the importance of undergraduate preparation, trainee selection, basic science education (particularly anatomy and pathology) postgraduate courses and supervised clinical experience. He also advocated the establishment of a minimum postgraduate training time for qualification in otolaryngology. Skillern, writing in the Journal of the American Medical Association (JAMA) in 'Post-graduate Work in Laryngology', echoed these concerns, noting that 'prior to 1918, practically no undergraduate teaching on a systematic and comprehensive scale had been successfully carried out in this country'.[8] Skillern observed that 'the aspiring young laryngologist became of the opinion that once the submucous resection and the enucleation of the tonsil were mastered, he forthwith had become a full-fledged and competent specialist'.[8] At that time, a 6-week course was typical for specialty training in otolaryngology. He called for a more rigorous and longer training in otolaryngology, and instruction in subspecialty areas such as laryngology and otology.

In the years following these early papers devoted to education in laryngology, only a few authors returned to this important subject. Milligan[9] argued that there was insufficient time devoted to laryngology in the undergraduate medical school curriculum in Britain. Dean[10] devoted his 1925 ALA Presidential Address to the teaching on undergraduate laryngology, and Layton[11] addressed undergraduate laryngology and postgraduate education in 1940. In 1966, Alford[12] wrote an excellent review of the evolution of undergraduate and graduate medical training in the United States, the development of standards and quality control, and the effects of the evolving medical educational milieu on residency training in otolaryngology. Bailey[13] provided interesting insights into the early years of the introduction of laryngology as a component of otolaryngology training for medical students in the same issue of Laryngoscope in which Alford's article was published. More than 50 years later, the training of medical students in laryngology remains an important and challenging issue, as does the education of the general public on the importance of laryngological and related disorders; but they are beyond the scope of this chapter, which is devoted to postgraduate training in laryngology. Currently, Medline lists many articles that address training in otolaryngology. However, considering the historical importance of laryngology to the development of otolaryngology, it is surprising how little has been written about teaching this challenging subspecialty.

In addition to concerns about curricular issues, laryngologists have been interested in the many practical aspects of teaching clinical laryngology. For example, before the advent of video-monitored laryngoscopy, a variety of devices was conceived to allow trainees to see the larynx during examinations performed by their mentors. Most involved the use of mirrors, such as Lukens' demonstroscope[14] in 1929 and a device developed at the Mayo clinic around 1960 that attached a shortened laryngeal mirror to a headlight with a reflecting mirror.[15] It is also worth remembering that the laryngeal mirror itself was originally introduced as a training device, albeit for singers, by singing teacher, Manuel Garcia in 1854.[16] A great many other clever devices have been introduced before and since that time that have enhanced diagnosis, treatment, and training in laryngology.[17] As early as 1936, Francis LeJeune reported that 'the motion picture film has been found of inestimable value in teaching the younger student clinical pathology of the larynx.[18] LeJeune's fascinating report indicates that he not only recognized the educational value of motion pictures in teaching laryngoscopy and laryngeal surgery, but also that he learned from his studies. His careful observations of the larynx helped him to advocate 'carrying out sharp dissection with the laryngeal knife for the removal of the growth. Such a procedure usually ensures as smooth, straight cord when healed'.[18] Nevertheless, because of the cumbersome equipment, the delay necessary to develop the film, and the time-consuming nature of motion picture laryngoscopy, this technology was not used widely in laryngology clinics. However, in the late 1950s and early 1960s, von Leden and Moore established a voice clinic and used highspeed motion pictures extensively in clinical care and laryngeal research.[19–22] They also described the importance of television as a teaching device in otolaryngology.[19] The application of an operating microscope to direct laryngoscopy improved not only surgical management but also training. Tardy[23] was among the first to highlight the importance of combining the microscope with a color television camera, in his 1972 article 'Microscopic Laryngology: Teaching Techniques'. He advocated television display of laryngeal surgery for the purpose of enhancing training, by allowing everyone in the operating room to see what the surgeon was doing. In addition to describing the value of new technology (microscope-assisted laryngoscopy and color television monitoring), Tardy showed photo documentation of magnified laryngeal polyp resection, using techniques considerably more delicate than the 'stripping' technique popular at the time. This insightful article listed specifically the teaching value of televised microscopic laryngeal surgery and called for its use in residency programs. Although

PART I: EDUCATION

today Tardy's observations seem obvious, it should be remembered that at that time, some respected otolaryngologists and educational institutions still considered the microscope (television monitoring aside) superfluous even for mastoid surgery, let alone laryngoscopy; and it was still believed by many that laryngoscopy could be performed perfectly well while holding an unsuspended laryngoscope with one hand and using instruments only in the other. Tardy's work was an important early step forward towards improving both physician education and patient care. Even so, it took a long time to catch on. For example, at the University of Michigan, the first camera for the otolaryngology department's microscope was not purchased until 1978. Even then, it was ordered by Dr. A.C.D. Brown of the department of anesthesia so that the anesthesiologist could see the surgical field during mastoid surgery, rather than by the otolaryngology department to enhance otological and laryngeal training. In retrospect, such lengthy delay in acquiring television monitors from so venerable a training program seems hard to fathom. Hence, it behooves each of us entrusted with the training of young otolaryngologists to reflect upon whether we are guilty of perpetrating similar unfathomable delays at our own institutions today.

Since 1975 (in English in 1977), when Hirano[24] described the layered structure of the vocal fold, laryngology has enjoyed unprecedented growth. Great advances in our understanding of the anatomy and physiology of phonation have been paralleled by technological developments for voice quantification and outcomes assessment.[25] These advances have resulted in dramatic improvement in the standard of care for all patients with laryngological disorders,[26] and they have affected clinical care remarkably quickly, due largely to exceptional interdisciplinary collaboration. Stimulated by meetings such as the Voice Foundation's Annual Symposium on Care of the Professional Voice, founded by Wilbur James Gould, Hans von Leden, and others in 1972, laryngologists, speech pathologists, basic science researchers, singing teachers, acting teachers, performers, and others have worked together to advance knowledge and enhance patient care. They have developed a common language, posed questions of practical value in the clinic and studio, and developed an interdisciplinary paradigm for answering important questions through valid, reliable research. Much of this research has been reported at meetings of the ALA and of the American Broncho-Esophalogical Association (ABEA), the Voice Foundation symposia and dozens of other, similar meetings that have evolved over the last four decades. Because of the interdisciplinary nature of many of these meetings and research efforts, the collaborative, penetrating discussions that occur among professionals of different disciplines at such meetings, even the most esoteric scientific advances are promulgated quickly. Their practical importance is probed at the time of their presentation, and new discoveries are applied to patient care around the world within days after such meetings end.

While the sheer amount of new information, equipment, diagnostic and therapeutic approaches, and surgical advancements is exciting, it has also created inconsistencies among training programs in the United States and throughout the world. Advances have been integrated piecemeal into various educational programs at different rates and to different degrees. Now that laryngology and voice is well established as a subspecialty, it seems timely to reflect on what we have learned, what anyone finishing a residency or a fellowship in laryngology and voice should be expected to know, and how we can best teach these essentials. The development and adoption of training guidelines for laryngology and voice should be encouraged not only to help program directors, but also to ensure reasonable consistency in minimal basic knowledge among graduates from all programs, with the end result being a consistently high level of care for laryngological patients. However, the rapid and successful evolution of our field highlights the need to consider more than just facts and skills as we develop training priorities. We should also try to impart an enthusiasm for the kind of interdisciplinary creativity that was responsible for our current evolution as a field and try to encourage and inspire similar academic and clinical creativity.

Residency training

While laryngology (including voice, speech, swallowing, airway and related disorders) constitutes only one segment of otolaryngology, it is particularly important for several reasons. First, laryngological problems are common. Estimates of the incidence of voice disorders in school-age children range, for example, from 6% to 23%.[27] Although there are few reliable, valid data on the incidence of voice disorders in the adult population, they are probably as prevalent as they are in children; and they may be even more common in elderly adults, who are more likely to develop neurological disorders with related voice, speech, and swallowing abnormalities. Most of our graduates will be called upon to care for patients with laryngological disorders and to educate colleagues (including primary care physicians) on the proper diagnosis and treatment of laryngeal problems. Second, the standard of care and state of the art have changed dramatically and continuously since the 1980s.[26,28] The diagnostic techniques, methods of documentation, and imperatives for outcomes assessment that are taken for granted now, were nonexistent just a few years ago. Some surgical techniques that were routine in the 1970s are now considered negligent, and newer surgical techniques that replaced them are already obsolete. If we do not make a concerted effort to ensure that our residents are fully aware of these developments and their practical implications, then they may provide outdated treatment; and both they and their patients will suffer the consequences.

Providing such training is especially difficult in laryngology because of the speed with which the field has developed. It is certainly not possible for all otolaryngologists, or even all academic otolaryngologists, to keep up with all developments in all fields within our specialty. There are many programs in which laryngology is managed and taught by general otolaryngologists, or by head and neck cancer surgeons without special training in the modern clinical and research aspects of laryngology. However, even if every training program in the United States had the desire and funds to hire an experienced and/or fellowship-trained laryngologist, there are not enough to supply all of the positions, yet. Therefore, at least until the number of laryngologists has caught up with the number needed, we must be especially diligent about defining expected areas of basic knowledge.

Details of a recommended curriculum are beyond the scope of this chapter. However, suggestions have been articulated, at least in preliminary form. One such document was developed by the Speech, Voice and Swallowing Committee of the American Academy of Otolaryngology, and another was developed by the American Laryngological Association (ALA). However, to date, no proposal has been accepted by the bodies that guide otolaryngology residency training.

The thoughts that follow constitute only a broad overview of this author's vision of minimum residency requirements with regard to substantive knowledge and clinical skill. They are offered not as definitive recommendations, but rather, to encourage continued dialog and an eventual consensus. This chapter concentrates on voice, because voice is the most advanced and complex division of laryngology at present, and in order to limit the length of this chapter. A similar model should be applied to training in the management of swallowing disorders, as well as selected speech-language disorders.

Basic science

Comprehensive knowledge of relevant anatomy, physiology, and pathology is required for insightful diagnosis and expert treatment of laryngological patients. Every trainee should be familiar with the layered microanatomy of the vocal fold, the characteristics of its basement membrane, neuromuscular anatomy (including the latest concepts in fiber composition and subspecialization within given muscles), laryngeal aging (from embryo to death), and the nature and importance of supraglottic and infraglottic components of the vocal tract. Neurolaryngology has emerged as a field and is vitally important to the clinician.[29] Just as neurotology has expanded our scope of training in otology, so must neurolaryngology in laryngology. Training should include elements of neuroanatomy and neurophysiology that seemed irrelevant until recently. Every graduate of a residency should also be familiar with the intricacies of voice physiology, including respiration, infraglottic power-source functions, the details of sound production at the level of the vocal folds, and the resonator functions of the supraglottic vocal tract. Understanding each component of the anatomy and physiology is not simply an academic exercise. Such knowledge allows the clinician to perform a 'systems analysis' on the voice, determine which components are malfunctioning or misfunctioning and establish diagnoses and treatment paradigms rationally.[28] Moreover, just as we expect our trainees to understand audiograms and how to interpret them, every trainee should be familiar with instrumentation for objective voice quantification and should be able to interpret data generated from voice laboratories. They also should be familiar with instruments for quality of life and outcomes assessments in patients with voice disorders.[30]

Research

Research is an essential component of any postgraduate training program. Ultimately, at its best, research is the means by which we figure out how to improve the condition of patients whom we cannot help now. Each resident should receive training in research methodology and should have practical experience with basic and/or clinical research. Such training is essential not only to teach incisive interpretation of the literature, but moreover to develop the ability to formulate precise questions relevant to the practice of laryngology, and to design rational paths toward their answers. Good research training should help solidify the dissatisfaction all physicians should feel about our limitations, and it should encourage a lifelong curiosity and an unwillingness to accept the limitations of our knowledge. Research should become a vital tool of daily practice through which we advance the boundaries of our specialty and enhance the care of our patients.

Diagnosis and medical management

Residents should master the details of the comprehensive, multisystem history required for patients with voice disorders, with special techniques for physical examination, and be familiar with the many other special considerations that must be taken into account when caring for voice professionals.[31-34] They should be able to recognize not only obvious laryngological problems, such as benign and malignant vocal fold lesions, but also less obvious lesions and related disorders. Graduates of our residencies should be able to differentiate voice dysfunctions emanating from the infraglottic or supraglottic vocal tract, as well as laryngeal manifestations of systemic disease (reflux, thyroid disease, and many others).[35] They should also gain experience in performing and interpreting strobovideolaryngoscopy and be familiar with the application of other diagnostic tests, including acoustic analysis, airflow assessment, laryngeal electromyography, high-speed video, and others. In addition, otolaryngology residents should receive specific training in the principles and practice of voice therapy, and they should spend at least some time observing therapy performed by an expert speech-language pathologist. Sufficient knowledge should be imparted to allow a laryngologist to determine whether a speech-language pathologist is providing his or her patient with appropriate, safe and beneficial therapy. Physicians who refer their patients to speech-language pathologists cannot fulfill this basic obligation unless they have a reasonable understanding of the indications for referral, of the techniques utilized by modern voice therapists and of the expected duration and progress of therapy. Ideally, residents also should be given an opportunity to work with a multidisciplinary voice team. It is also essential, of course, for trainees to be familiar with medical treatment, including the vocal consequences of various medical treatment of voice disorders prescribed by otolaryngologists and other physicians (iatrogenic dysphonias).

In addition, we must prepare for our trainees for 'special situations' - for example, complex problems such as laryngeal trauma, vocal fold scarring and arytenoid cartilage dislocations that often require special expertise and/or rapid diagnosis and management. High-performance professional voice users also pose special challenges, obligations and risks with which any practicing otolaryngologist should be familiar in order to avoid well-meaning but potentially costly treatment errors.

Surgery

Otolaryngology boasts an excellent tradition of teaching surgical skills. Prior to performing neck surgery on humans, residents have been instructed on the anatomy and physiology of neck structures and pathophysiology and they have performed neck dissection on cadavers. Generally, they also have observed or assisted in numerous similar surgical procedures. The training tradition is even more consistent and rigorous for surgery of the temporal bone. Temporal bone laboratory dissection with professional instruction and supervision is required in most programs before residents are entrusted with surgical care of human ears. Unfortunately, the same systematic approach to teaching of surgical skills is often not applied to laryngeal surgery in most institutions. Laryngeal endoscopy, microscopic voice surgery, and phonosurgery (including framework surgery) are amenable to a similar thorough and systematic approach to training. In addition to instruction in anatomy and physiology of phonation, examination and quantification of voice function, outcomes assessment, alternatives to surgery and timing of surgery before operating, the resident should have a thorough knowledge of surgical instrumentation (traditional and laser). Practice under supervision in laryngeal dissection laboratories (similar to temporal bone laboratories) and periods of observation in the operating room should precede resident surgery on human larynges. Attention to surgical technique and ergonomics is essential, because of the technical difficulties involved in maintaining perfect control of the tips of long laryngeal instruments. Laryngeal microsurgery may well be approached conceptually as ear surgery with longer instruments. Resident surgery on patients should be supervised closely and should follow a planned progression from simple to complex cases; and it should be recognized that microdissection of the vibratory margin of the vocal fold may be more challenging technically than some seemingly 'larger' cases such as laryngectomy. Results from residents' surgery should be comparable to those achieved by professorial faculty. Training also should include criteria for determining which cases should not be performed by the inexperienced or occasional laryngeal surgeon, and guidelines for referral to tertiary care laryngologists.

Special considerations

In addition to providing training in facts and skills, attention must be paid to the art of patient care. This is extremely important in the management of all patients, and especially so when caring for high-performance voice professionals.

Residents in otolaryngology, and fellows in laryngology and voice, should be imbued with curiosity about the many questions that remain unanswered. They should receive historical information about the developments of our field, and exposure to voice professionals in other disciplines, such as speech-language pathologists, singing voice specialists, and arts-medicine specialists in other fields.

Fellowship training

Fellowship programs in laryngology have proliferated in response to clinical and academic demand, but they have actually existed for many years. For example, the late Dr. Hans von Leden and the late Dr. Wilbur James Gould trained fellows starting in the 1950s and 1960s, among them such distinguished individuals as Drs. Minoru Hirano and Nobuhiko Isshiki. This author began providing such training in 1981 and, since that time, our fellows have included not only laryngologists, but also speech-language pathologists, singing teachers and others. If our specialty is to provide enough practitioners to meet the need for high-caliber laryngology and voice care teams, then we must participate in training for physicians and for professionals in other disciplines who will constitute the interdisciplinary teams of the future.

While no formal guidelines for fellowship training have been accepted universally, a document developed by Dr. Robert Ossoff, this author, and other members of the Ad Hoc Committee on Laryngology Fellowship of the ALA has provided a useful framework and can be accessed through the ALA's website. The need for quality control and some standardization in minimum experience in fellowship programs will hopefully lead to further action and ongoing revision of this document or a similar set of guidelines.

Creative thought

Interdisciplinary opportunities for creativity in medicine still offer the potential for excitement, joy, and innovation in daily practice.[36] The current advances in laryngology were inspired by interest in the problems of professional voice users, particularly opera singers; but this trend in laryngology was not isolated. Modern voice medicine is but one component of a larger field of arts medicine that offers similar interdisciplinary team care for pianists, string players, dancers, wind instrumentalists, and others.[37] The arts-medicine aspects of laryngology are exciting for at least two reasons that should be addressed in any training program. First, performers and artists place critical demands on their bodies, and they do not have the usual tolerance for incomplete cures. An injured finger that returns to 98% normal function and is adequate for a microsurgeon, might not be adequate for a premier violinist. That extra 2% separates the famous artist from the local violin teacher. Arts-medicine patients force us to redefine 'normal' much more narrowly, and they challenge our abilities to recognize, quantify, and restore physiological perfection. Much of the fun and many of the ideas that have helped advance laryngology and voice have come from close interactions with such patients, as well as with speech-language pathologists, voice scientists, singing teachers, acting teachers, and other colleagues, all of whom provide insights useful in clinical practice. Second, arts medicine provides physicians with an opportunity to work closely with professionals and educators in the arts and humanities. The arts and medicine are inherently similar in many ways. However, through our educational process, physicians too often lose sight of the importance of the arts to our practices. Arts medicine offers the clinician a chance to work and think with colleagues, such as artists and performers, and to find new solutions to complex problems. It might even inspire us to study one of the arts. As we strive to master the science and art of healing, our colleagues in the arts and humanities can help expand insight, sensitivity and ability to empathize. Such interactions also help keep us from being trapped intellectually by existing paradigms and allow us to approach questions with a broader vision, creating new solutions to problems that seem insurmountable within the compartmentalized framework of our traditional training - and even allow us to create new fields of medicine.

Conclusion

Laryngologists of the future will ideally be positioned to thrive as sophisticated diagnosticians, surgeons and scientists; but they also will have exceptional opportunities to remain 'physicians' in the truest and broadest sense. It is incumbent upon us to offer training environments that will not merely provide skills, but also will kindle and nurture their curiosity, creativity and broadest vision. In these days of economic and legal crises, medicine has precious few reminders of the reasons why most of us were inspired to become doctors. For the last four decades, modern laryngology has been built on such enthusiasm, and practicing it remains exhilarating. We must ensure that the next generation will not have to settle for anything less. If we are successful, 20 years from now, our practice will look as crude as Elsberg's methods seem to us now; and we will have accomplished our mission as educators and left behind training centers filled not only with information, but also with inspiration and imagination.

References

1. Elsberg L. Presidential Address to the First Meeting of the American Laryngological Association. *Trans Am Laryngol Assoc* 1879;1:33–90.
2. Elsberg L. Presidential Address to the Second Meeting of the American Laryngological Association. *Trans Am Laryngol Assoc* 1880;2:3–11.
3. Knight F. Presidential Address to the Fourth Meeting of the American Laryngological Association. *Trans Am Laryngol Assoc* 1882;4:2–11.
4. Wilders JSS. On the teaching on Laryngology. *Br Med J* 1890;2:376–77.
5. Swain HL. Laryngology and its place in medical education: Presidential Address to the Twenty-Third Meeting of the American Laryngological Association. *Trans Am Laryngol Assoc* 1901;23:1–17.
6. Knight CH. The teaching of laryngology, then and now. *Laryngoscope* 1906;160:840–43.

7. Harris TJ. The training of the specialist. *Ann Otolo Rhinol Laryngol* 1913;22:475–81.
8. Skillern RH. Post-graduate work in laryngology. *JAMA* 1921;77:1145–46.
9. Milligan W. The rise and progress of laryngology: its relation to general medicine and its position in the medical curriculum. *Br Med J* 1922;1:547–51.
10. Dean LW. The teaching of undergraduate laryngology. *Laryngoscope* 1925;35:735–41.
11. Layton TB. The aims and methods of teaching laryngology. *J Laryngol Otol* 1940;55:495–502.
12. Alford BR. The age of the medical education revolution. *Laryngoscope* 1966;106:801–4.
13. Bailey BJ. Laryngology education at the turn of the century. *Laryngoscope* 1966;106:797–800.
14. Ridpath RF. Diseases of the larynx. In: Jackson C, Coates GM. Eds. *The nose, throat, and ear and their diseases*. Philadelphia, Pennsylvania: WB Saunders, 1929:736–44.
15. Shahrokh DK, Devine KD. A teaching device for residents in laryngology. *Arch Otolaryngol* 1961;74:234–5.
16. Garcia M. Observations on the human voice. *Proc R Soc Lond* 1855;7:397–410.
17. Zeitels SM. Premalignant epithelium and microinvasive cancer of the vocal fold: the evolution of phonomicrosurgical management. *Laryngoscope* 1995;105(suppl 67).
18. LeJeune FE. Motion picture study of laryngeal lesions. *Surg Gynecol Obstet* 1936;62:492–5.
19. Moore P, von Leden H. Television in otolaryngology and other specialties. A new teaching device. *JAMA* 1959;169:1976–80.
20. von Leden H. Laryngeal physiology: cinematographic observations. *J Laryngol Otol* 1960;74:705–12.
21. Moore GP, White FD, von Leden H. Ultra high speed photography in laryngeal physiology. *J Speech Hear Disord* 1962;27:162–71.
22. von Leden H, Le Cover M, Ringel RL, Isshiki N. Improvements in laryngeal cinematography. *Arch Otolaryngol* 1966;83:482–87.
23. Tardy ME. Microscopic laryngology: teaching techniques. *Laryngoscope* 1972;82:1315–22.
24. Hirano M. Structure and vibratory pattern of the vocal folds. In: Sawashima N, Cooper FS. Eds. *Dynamic aspects of speech production*. Tokyo, Japan: University of Tokyo Press 1977:13–24.
25. Sataloff RT. The human voice. *Sci Am* 1992;267:108–15.

26. Sataloff RT. *Professional Voice: The Science and Art of Clinical Care*, 4th Ed. San Diego, California: Plural Publishing, Inc., 2017.
27. National strategic research plan of the National Institute on Deafness and Other Communication Disorders, 1991, 1992, 1993. NIH Publication #95–3711. Bethesda, MD: US Department of Health and Human Services, 1995:270.
28. Sataloff RT. Rational Thought: the impact of voice science upon voice care. *J Voice* 1995;9:215–34.
29. Sataloff RT. *Neurolaryngology*. San Diego, California: Plural Publishing, Inc., 2017.
30. Benninger MS, Syamal MN, Gardner GM, Jacobson BH. New directions in measuring voice treatment outcomes and quality of life. In: Sataloff RT. *Professional Voice: The Science and Art of Clinical Care*, 4th Ed. San Diego, California: Plural Publishing, Inc., 2017:547–58.
31. Sataloff RT. Patient History. In: Sataloff RT. *Professional Voice: The Science and Art of Clinical Care*, 4th Ed. San Diego, California: Plural Publishing, Inc., 2017:363–86.
32. Raphael BN. Special Considerations relating to members of the acting profession. In: Sataloff RT. *Professional Voice: The Science and Art of Clinical Care*, 4th Ed. San Diego, California: Plural Publishing, Inc., 2017:387–90.
33. Sataloff RT. Physical examination. In: Sataloff RT. *Professional Voice: The Science and Art of Clinical Care*, 4th Ed. San Diego, California: Plural Publishing, Inc., 2017:391–404.
34. Romak JJ, Heuer R, Hawkshaw MJ, Sataloff RT. The clinical voice laboratory. In: Sataloff RT. *Professional Voice: The Science and Art of Clinical Care*, 4th Ed. San Diego, California: Plural Publishing, Inc., 2017:405–38.
35. Hamdan A, Sataloff RT, Hawkshaw MJ *Laryngeal Manifestations of Systemic Diseases*. San Diego, California: Plural Publishing, Inc., 2018, in press.
36. Sataloff RT. Interdisciplinary opportunities for creativity in medicine. *ENT J* 1998;77:530–3.
37. Sataloff RT, Brandfonbrener A, Lederman R, eds. *Performing Arts Medicine*, 3rd ed. Narberth, Pennsylvania: Science and Medicine, 2010.

Reprinted with modifications by permission of SAGE Publications from:
Sataloff RT. Education in Laryngology: Rising to Old Challenges. *Ann Otol Rhinol Laryngol* 1999;108(11):1046–52.

11. World Voice Day

World Voice Day is celebrated annually and is described in this chapter. In addition to its intrinsic merit, this event might serve as an excellent model to highlight health issues in other disciplines throughout the day. All physicians, speech-language pathologists, singing and acting teachers, performers voice patients and others who care for and about the voice are encouraged to work together to raise awareness of the importance of the voice and of developments in voice care.

The World Health Organization recognized a particularly high rate of laryngeal cancer in Brazil. In April 1989, Brazilian otolaryngologists established a National Voice Week. Soon, other societies around the world recognized the importance of public education about the voice; and the European Laryngological Association (www.elsoc.org), American Bronchoesophagological Association (www.abea.net), and other societies began collaborating an annual World Voice Day.

World Voice Day was celebrated in the United States for the first time on April 16, 2003. It was supported by the American Academy of Otolaryngology–Head and Neck Surgery (AAO-HNS) (www.entnet.org), the Voice Foundation (www.voicefoundation.org), the American Laryngological Association (www.alahns.org), and numerous other societies and organizations. A summary of the evolution of World Voice Day can be found on the website of the American Academy of Otolaryngology-Head and Neck Surgery at www.entnet.org. and at WorldVoiceDay.org.

Typical World Voice Day activities include free voice screenings, lectures, concerts, educational programs, and media events scheduled to take place on April 16th and, often, for a few days surrounding that date. Web-based educational initiatives may be found through the AAO-HNS website and elsewhere. Laryngologists, speech-language pathologists, nurses, singers, singing teachers, actors, acting teachers and others organize celebratory events in cities throughout the world. They are bound together by a commitment to expand public appreciation of and knowledge about the human voice, and to raise awareness about the importance of good vocal health and education.

For example, in Philadelphia in 2018, World Voice Day events included free clinical voice screenings, a PECO (Philadelphia Electric Company) Crown Lights display visible throughout much of the city, voice education presentations, and a concert. In other years, activities also have included readings by authors of children's books to Philadelphia school children (with introductions about vocal health), vocal health workshops, master classes, comedy club presentations featuring vocal versatility, presentations by storytellers and other events that highlight to the public the importance and fragility of the human voice.

Extensive events honoring World Voice Day take place each year in Lisbon, Portugal under the auspices of Professor Mario Andrea, in the Detroit area under the guidance of Dr. Adam Rubin, in Pittsburgh with Dr. Libby Smith; in Los Angeles under the guidance of Dr. Michael Johns; in San Francisco under the leadership of Dr. Clark Rosen; in Cleveland guided by Dr. Michael Benninger; and in many other cities. In addition, the US National Association of Teachers of Singing supports World Voice Day actively, and many events around the country, indeed the world, are organized by singing teachers.

Future activities promise to be even more expansive as guided through the new ad hoc World Voice Day planning committee, notable for its broad international representation. The group's initial meeting was held in Erlangen, Germany, on July 4, 2012; and the organization is committed to sharing the excitement of voice science, pedagogy and the vocal arts globally in collaboration with like-minded existing groups. Under the guidance initially of Johan Sundberg, Ph.D., in Stockholm, Sweden, and recently also of Dr. Mara Behlau, this group documented 461 World Voice Day events in 2014, 736 in 2016, and 632 in 2017 (when April 16th was on Easter Sunday), and continuing growth thereafter. The WorldVoiceDay.org website is functioning as an historical and current repository of World Voice Day events globally with pivotal key personnel in 65 countries; and major organizations (including the American Academy of Otolaryngology–Head and Neck Surgery and The Voice Foundation) are collaborating with that initiative.

To assist with the educational mission of World Voice Day, the AAO-HNS developed a website, fact sheets on common voice problems, and materials for press releases to assist local communities in developing Word Voice Day events. These materials are updated regularly and are available through the Academy. The Academy also establishes annual World Voice Day themes for the American celebration. In the past, these have included 'Listen to your voice, it might be telling you something', 'Put your best voice forward', 'Don't tax your voice', 'Invest in your voice', 'Love your voice', 'Voice: The Original Social Media', 'Explore your voice', and 'Share your voice'.

World Voice Day is still not acknowledged actively in too many communities throughout the world. This occasion offers an opportunity for all voice care professionals to collaborate with each other, bringing together colleagues in otolaryngology, speech-language pathology, singing, acting, public speaking, education, the media, and other occupations. Vocal health is critical to our communication-oriented society, but the voice does not receive the public recognition, appreciation or funding that it deserves. World Voice Day provides a perfect forum through which to re-familiarize ourselves with the latest advances in laryngology and voice care, and to educate our colleagues, patients, and communities via lectures, free voice screenings, community outreach programs, and other offerings.

Extraordinary advances in voice diagnosis and treatment have elevated the standard of care for voice patients throughout the world. World Voice Day provides a perfect opportunity to share these advances with our professional colleagues, the general public, and the media. We are justly proud of advances in the state-of-the-art of voice care over the past few decades. Generating increased awareness and interest within the public will not only bring the availability of modern voice care to the attention of more people, but it also might help engender the kind of public enthusiasm and support needed to facilitate even greater advances in the future.

Reprinted with modifications by permission of Vendome Group from:
Sataloff RT. World Voice Day 2016. *ENT J* 2016;95(3):92–5.

12. The otolaryngology residency application problem

The challenges of gaining acceptance to an otolaryngology residency are familiar not only to those of us in academics, but also to anyone who has tried to help a medical student gain entrance to one of our training programs. The pressures and cost of applying to otolaryngology residency are increasing, and the large number of applications submitted by each applicant makes it challenging for residency programs to figure out who is really interested in a specific institution.

In August 2016, Wong proposed a solution that involved organizing residency programs into consortia, based on similar characteristics such as geography and a supported research year.[1] Graboyes and Goebel offered commentary and critique on the same issue.[2] We can always count on Joel Goebel and his group for thoughtful insights and that commentary is no exception.

Graboyes and Goebel enumerated potential problems with Wong's innovative suggestion. The critiques included bias that might be created in residency reputation based on exclusion from consortia, or self-exclusion from consortia by elite programs; bias against residents who applied but were not invited for interviews by consortia for early match (the consortia concept provided for early match, with those failing to match entering the current National Resident Matching Program [NRMP] match); problems in choosing meaningful criteria on which to base the aggregation of programs into consortia; challenges in selecting the best candidates for invitation

PART I: EDUCATION

to interview for a consortia match; and the likelihood that the NRMP would not allow such a system.

Both Wong and his critics raise valid concerns, but the problems remain unsolved.

The Society of University Otolaryngologists-Head and Neck Surgeons and the Association of Academic Departments of Otolaryngology-Head and Neck Surgery are sensitive to the problems facing our applicants and discuss them routinely. Electronic residency application service data revealed that there was a median of 32 applications per applicant in 2017.[3] Those data also revealed that in 2016, otolaryngology residency applicants who were members of Alpha Omega Alpha (AOA) submitted a median of 59 applications for otolaryngology residency, and in 2017 they submitted 54. The costs associated with each application include not only monitory requirements but also time and stress.

Suggestions for easing this situation have included limiting the number of applications permitted,[4] using standardized letters of recommendation,[5-7] guiding otolaryngology program directors to counsel students to apply to a carefully chosen group of 10 to 20 programs,[8,9] and requiring that a portion of each personal statement include specific information about why the applicant is interested in that specific program. In my opinion, while all these suggestions have merit, they also have shortcomings.

For example, forcibly limiting the number of applications that an applicant is permitted to submit not only seems somewhat contrary to the basic principles of freedom of choice, but it also has potential disadvantages for both applicants and programs. Setting aside the difficulty of figuring out how to select the correct number of programs at which to set the limit, limiting the number of applications could potentially hurt not only weaker applicants, but also the strongest. Weaker applicants probably would be forced to eliminate most or all their 'reach' programs. This would be troublesome not only for the applicants, but also for the programs.

We have all seen students who were not our best applicants on paper do so well on 'away rotations' that they were accepted into and thrived in elite programs that no one would have predicted would take them. Not only have such training opportunities benefited the applicants, but the applicants also often have provided diversity that strengthened the programs. If the number of applications were limited, these applicants probably would not 'waste' away rotations at programs that they deemed unlikely to accept them.

Program directors and otolaryngology medical student advisors already should be advising applicants to focus on a relatively small number of programs that are their top choices, selected from programs at which they appear competitive. I advise my students to select their top 3 to 5 choices and an additional 10 to 15 at which they would be happy. However, while they choose their away rotations and focus their efforts on these programs, they all know there is no guarantee that they will be accepted to one of them, and they apply to many more. In the current system, I would not advise them to do otherwise. So, this approach alone will not decrease the number of applications.

Much can be said in favor of standardized letters of recommendation. However, although they have been discussed for several years, they have yet to be adopted uniformly in otolaryngology, and opinions and experiences in other specialties vary.[10-13] Moreover, unless these standardized letters include or are supplemented by free-form commentary, much of the most valuable, personal information about applicants might not be conveyed well enough. In addition, it seems unlikely that this approach will reduce the number of applications per candidate.

Many applicants already have been writing paragraphs within their personal statements that are specific to each program. For a few years, that was required; but the requirement has been dropped and such program-specific paragraphs are optional for most residencies. While program directors certainly read such statements, they also know they may be written for each program and might be pro forma, and that might hamper the credibility of the program-specific paragraph.

So, we have medical students applying to an oppressive number of programs, and programs receiving a burdensome number of applications from which it is often difficult to cull applicants with a genuine interest in any specific institution. I do not have a perfect solution, but I have a thought for a simple approach that might help.

The matching program was instituted for good reasons, including protecting applicants from being placed under undue pressure. I am personally familiar with the old system. At the end of my first day of an away rotation at the Massachusetts Eye and Ear Infirmary, I received a phone call and was given 10 seconds to accept or decline a residency position at the University of Michigan. I accepted gratefully, but I would not have minded the option (which I requested and was denied) to defer that decision until I had spent a month at Harvard. Nevertheless, there seems to be room for a happy medium between the old, unregulated system and the current, richly regulated NRMP.

For example, in college admissions, early-decision programs work well. Students who are accepted are spared the arduous task of applying to multiple colleges in which they are less interested, and colleges can select from applicants whom they know are committed to their institution. Applying early decision to one college has no demonstrated adverse effect on applications at other colleges; and people who are rejected during the early-decision process commonly are accepted to their early-decision school later during the regular application process.

While a similar early-application option for otolaryngology residency would not solve all of our problems, it is a simple, time-tested approach that might help, especially if it were timed with an ample period between the decision and the match-application deadline, so that early-decision applicants would not have to fill out their 60 additional applications and wait to 'push the button' in case they were rejected from their early-decision program.

Since there is so much academic precedent for early-decision models, it seems possible that the NRMP would be willing to discuss such an option, with the early-decision program either separate from and well before the match, or possibly administered through the match. If 20% of residency positions were filled by early decision, assuming many of these candidates would be AOA-level applicants, that would not only put those students into their first-choice programs and help programs fill with applicants who really want to be there, but it also would decrease by about 3,600 the number of applications through which other programs had to sift.

Early decision is only one simple, partial solution to the problem of excessive applications. There are undoubtedly others. However, it seems clear that it is time for us to not just think about this issue, but also to act. We have recognized for years the difficulties that the current system poses for applicants and programs. It is past time to start improving our system.

References

1. Wong BJ. Reforming the match process-early decision plans and the case for a consortia match. *JAMA Otolaryngol HNS* 2016;142(8):727–8.
2. Graboyes EM, Goebel JA. Reforming the otolaryngology-head and neck surgery match: Should we embrace a consortia match? *JAMA Otolaryngol HNS* 2016;142(8):728–30.
3. Association of American Medical Colleges. Otolaryngology: using ERAS since ERAS 2006. https://www.aamc.org/download/358802/data/otolaryngology.pdf. Published 2017. Accessed August 20, 2018.
4. Naclerio RM, Pinto JM, Baroody FM. Drowning in applications for residency training: A program's perspective and simple solutions. *JAMA Otolaryngol HNS* 2014;140(8):695–6.
5. Perkins JN, Liang C, McFann K, et al. Standardized letter of recommendation for otolaryngology residency selection. *Laryngoscope* 2013;123(1):123–33.
6. Messner A, Teng M, Shimahara E, et al. A case for the standardized letter of recommendation in otolaryngology residency selection. *Laryngoscope* 2014:124(1):2–3.

7. Kominsky AH, Bryson PC, Benninger MS, Tierney WS. Variability of ratings in the otolaryngology standardized letter of recommendation. *Otolaryngol HNS* 2016;154(2):287–93.
8. Baroody FM, Pinto JM, Naclerio RM. Otolaryngology (urban) legend: The more programs to which you apply, the better the chances of matching. *Arch Otolaryngol HNS* 2008;134(10):1038.
9. Christophel JJ, Levine PA. Too much of a good thing. *JAMA Otolaryngol HNS* 2014;140(4):291–2.
10. Nallasamy S, Uhler T, Nallasamy N, et al. Ophthalmology resident selection: Current trends in selection criteria and improving the process. *Ophthalmology* 2010;117(8):1505.
11. Diab J, Riley S, Overton DT. The Family Education Rights and Privacy Act's impact on residency applicant behavior and recommendations: A pilot study. *J Emerg Med* 2011;40(1):72–5.
12. Love JN, Deiorio NM, Ronan-Bentle S, et al. SLOR Task Force. Characterization of the Council of Emergency Medicine Residency Directors' standardized letter of recommendation in 2011-2012. *Acad Emerg Med* 2013;20(9):926–32.
13. Diab J, Riley S, Downes A, et al. A multicenter study of the family educational rights and privacy act and the standardized letter of recommendation: Impact on emergency medicine residency applicant and faculty behaviors. *J Grad Med Educ* 2014;6(2):292–5.

Reprinted with modifications by permission of Vendome Group from:
Sataloff RT. The otolaryngology residency application problem. *ENT J* 2017;96(3):91–3.

13. Interviews: Less helpful than we think, or harmful

Like many of us, I always have placed considerable value on interviews for student applicants, potential residents, attendings interested in joining my practice and faculty, and staff. An article in the *New York Times* (sent to me by a friend who subscribes) has led me to reconsider the usefulness of a process that I assumed had 'obvious' value.

In 2017, Jason Dana, an Assistant Professor of Management and Marketing at the Yale School of Management, published an article in the *New York Times*.[1] A computer search for articles that he has produced revealed a preliminary discussion published in 2012, on the University of Pennsylvania website[2], and a peer-reviewed paper that reported the final results of that study. Dana's research and insights are both interesting and somewhat disturbing.[3]

As educators and employers, most of us use free-form, unstructured interviews. We believe that they give us a good idea of a person, whether we are interviewing a job candidate or an applicant for medical school, residency, or another position. Dana's observations suggest that we 'typically form strong but unwarranted impressions about interviewees'[1], often revealing more about ourselves than the candidates. Several examples highlight the kinds of errors that result from job interviews.

Dana[1] described a case of a friend who believed that she had arrived five minutes early for a job interview, had a pleasant and friendly discussion with the interviewers, and was offered the job. After the interview, it was learned that the interviewers had been impressed that she was so composed after showing up 25 minutes late for the interview. Actually, she had been told the wrong start time and had no idea that she was late for the interview. If she had been, it is unlikely that she would have behaved as comfortably as she had. Consequently, the decision to hire her based on the assumption that her behavior in the interview indicated her future job performance under pressure was fundamentally flawed.

Dana also recounted an interesting anecdote from the University of Texas medical school at Houston from 1979. Late in the student selection season, the medical school was ordered by the Legislature to increase its incoming class size by 50 students. The additional students who were accepted to fill those 50 seats had reached the interview phase, but following their interviews they had been rejected. Later research showed no difference in terms of academic performance, clinical performance (including human interaction), honors earned and attrition between those 50 students and the rest of the class who had had successful interviews leading to admission.

Dana argues that his research indicates that interviews are not merely irrelevant, but moreover are harmful, undercutting the value of more valuable information about interviewees. He and his co-authors had students interview other students and attempt to predict grade point averages for the following semester based on the interview, the student's course schedule, and his/her past grade point average (GPA)[3]. The researchers explained in advance that past GPA was the best predictor of future grades at their school. The students who participated in the research also were asked to predict the performance of students whom they did not meet, based solely on the students' course schedules and past GPAs. The results showed that the GPA predictions were significantly more accurate for students they did not meet, and that the interviews had been counterproductive. In addition, the researchers had introduced interviewees who had been instructed to respond randomly to interview questions. In half of the interviews, interviewees were instructed to answer honestly, and the other half were instructed to answer randomly using a specific formula and responding to a group of yes/no or this/that questions. It was fascinating to note that not a single interviewer noticed that he/she was conducting an interview with random answers; and all the students who unwittingly conducted random interviews rated the degree to which they got to know the interviewee slightly higher on average than those who conducted honest interviews. Dana observed that "the key psychological insight here is that people have no trouble turning any information into a coherent narrative.... People can't help seeing signals, even in noise."[1]

In a fascinating sequel, the researchers explained what they had done, including their findings, to another group of student subjects. Thereafter, they asked them what information they would like to have in order to make a GPA prediction. They all still wanted interviews, believing that, despite the data, they would be able to glean useful information from personal interviews on which to base their predictions.

Most of us think that we can learn something useful from personal interviews, usually unstructured, but Dana believes that we are wrong. He recognizes that unstructured interviews will continue but advises that we be very conservative in the interpretations and conclusions we draw from them. He also recommends that structured interviews, with all candidates receiving the same questions, provide better information, as do interviews directed specifically to test job-related skills.

Whether we are interviewing potential secretaries, students, associates, hospital administrators, political candidates or others, most of us have considerable faith in our abilities to 'read people'. Perhaps we are not as good at doing so as we think. Clearly, the subject requires further research and maybe an extra dose of humility and circumspection.

References

1. Dana J. The Utter Uselessness of Job Interviews. *New York Times*, April 8, 2017. https://www.nytimes.com/2017/04/08/opinion/sunday/the-utter-uselessness-of-job-interviews.html?mcubz=1. Accessed on August 19, 2018.
2. Dana J, Dawes RM, Peterson NR. Belief in the Unstructured Interview: The Persistence of an Illusion. August 15, 2012. http://www.sas.upenn.edu/~danajd/interview.pdf Accessed on August 19, 2018.
3. Dana J, Dawes R, Peterson N. Belief in the unstructured interview: The persistence of an illusion. *Judgment and Decision Making* 2013;8:512-20.

Reprinted with modifications by permission of Vendome Group from:
    Sataloff RT. Interviews: less helpful than we think or harmful. ENT J, in press.

14. Hiring young doctors: What physicians should know about changes in the medical school curriculum

For decades, the medical school curriculum remained 'traditional'. Most of us received two years of basic science teaching followed by two years of clinical exposure. That model, which had been standard since about 1910, has changed in response to evolving needs in the healthcare environment. In order to prepare young doctors to meet the demands of America's rapidly changing healthcare system, medical schools have made major adjustments. It is helpful for physicians to understand some of these changes so that we can have realistic understanding and expectations of young doctors whom we recruit for residencies or our practices.

One of the fundamental shortcomings of our traditional approach to medical education has been the narrow focus on treating the physical disease of an individual patient, with little or no attention to public health implications. The Association of American Medical Colleges (AAMC) has stressed the importance of this problem for a few years and encouraged medical schools to address it through curricular change.[1] Many schools have responded. Students are being taught to view health problems not only focused on the individual, but moreover at a population level. Obvious public health issues that we should consider on a daily basis include prevention-related services, immunization, infection control and other topics. During the last decade, many medical schools have introduced progressively more public health content into the required medical school curriculum, and some facilitate certificates or masters degrees in public/population health for their medical students. For example, in Philadelphia, beginning with the class of 2014, the Sidney Kimmel Medical College of Thomas Jefferson University created a 'college within the college' program to provide students with academic and research options in areas of population health, in association with Jefferson's School of Population Health (as opposed to Public Health), founded in 2009 and the first of its kind. Many medical schools offer and encourage dual degree programs in medicine and public health. Students who graduate with such education bring a broader perspective on the implications of disease and medical care to our patients, departments and practices.

Medical schools have instituted other major changes to the traditional curriculum. In an increasing number of medical schools, the initial basic science training has been condensed from two years to one and a half years, or even one year. Most schools introduce clinical experience immediately, with student-patient contact starting within the first weeks of medical school. In some, additional basic science training is added to the curriculum in the latter years of medical school, after students have selected a specialty, so that they can concentrate their in-depth basic science studies in their areas of primary interest.

Some schools have introduced even more creative changes to help students gain a practical understanding of health care.[2] For example, at the Pennsylvania State College of Medicine in Hershey, students begin their medical training as patient navigators, helping patients and their families get through the medical system, and experiencing the confusions and frustrations of medical care firsthand, changing dramatically the students' practical understanding of the patient experience. This process also gives them exceptional exposure (physical and bureaucratic) to the health system in which they will train. At New York University, students track all hospital admissions and charges in the state. This leads to provocative discussions of the health care system and discrepancies in the care of different populations, such as the $3,000 the cost for delivering a baby in rural New York compared with the $22,000 cost for the same service in New York City. Students at Hofstra North Shore-Long Island Jewish School of Medicine do not spend their first two months in medical school lectures at all. Rather, they all become certified emergency medical technicians and experience firsthand the making of rapid, life-saving judgments through 911 calls. The Mayo Clinic medical school converted much of the material taught traditionally in didactic lecture classes to electronic format, allowing students to study it on their own time and to use class time for case studies and discussion. Mayo also added a four-year course called The Science of Healthcare Delivery that teaches biomedical informatics, systems engineering, and healthcare economics.

Even the admissions criteria for medical schools have changed. The medical college admission test (MCAT) is now 2 hours longer (6.5 hours) than the test most of us took. The added material includes questions on social and behavioral sciences, in addition to the standard information in chemistry, biology and physics. Among other things, the redesigned test encourages prospective medical students to have a broader education and perspective than one might get from concentrating solely on the facts needed to be a biology major.

In addition, many medical schools are decreasing emphasis on memorizing material. This may be partly because of the rapidity with which medical facts are changing, and partially because of the ubiquitous availability of electronic information. Rather, schools are teaching students to seek information efficiently and routinely, and to utilize technology.

Some schools are considering reducing the curriculum from four years to three years, allowing students to graduate and start residencies sooner. The AAMC is studying ways to use mastery of competencies as criteria for graduation rather than a specific number of years, allowing students to master information and skills at a pace of their choosing.

Like medical practice and healthcare delivery systems, medical education is evolving. Recent medical school graduates are undoubtedly trained as well as most of us were, but differently. It is helpful for physicians to recognize these differences in training as we work with residents or hire young associates. Such understanding might do more than alter our expectations and the way we interact with new physicians; it also might highlight the many things that we can learn from young doctors educated in the new paradigm.

References

1. Jablow M. The Public Health Imperative: Revising the Medical School Curriculum. AAMC, May 2015.
2. Beck M. Innovation is sweeping through U.S. medical schools. The Wall Street Journal, February 16, 2015. https://www.wsj.com/articles/innovation-is-sweeping-through-u-s-medical-schools-1424145650. Accessed on August 13, 2018.

Reprinted with modifications by permission of Vendome Group from:

Sataloff RT. Hiring Young Doctors: What Otolaryngologists Should Know About Changes in the Medical School Curriculum. ENT J, in press.

Part II: Research

15. HIPAA: An impediment to research

The Health Insurance Portability and Accountability Act (HIPAA), which became effective in the USA on April 14, 2003, was intended to help ensure patient privacy and to increase patients' control of their personal health information. However, implementation has created numerous practical problems. Many of these drawbacks are familiar to clinicians who have had to deal with increased costs and decreased efficiency of patient care, without obvious benefit to patient safety or privacy. Economic consequences of HIPAA were recognized promptly after it was implemented.[1] However, in addition to clinical and economic consequences, the adverse effects of HIPAA upon research should not be underestimated. These effects are particularly troublesome because of difficulties created by HIPAA in performing research based upon review of medical records.

Although retrospective chart reviews do not have the cachet of blinded, randomized, prospective research, they have been an important component of medical literature in the evolution of most medical specialties. For generations, residents and clinicians have reviewed clinical data retrospectively to assess outcomes, identify areas of success and failure, seek opportunities for improvement, and define questions that warrant prospective, randomized, controlled studies. For most of the 20th century, no institutional review board (IRB) approval was sought or expected for retrospective studies, especially since patients were not identified. More recently, most IRBs approved retrospective studies, waiving informed consent, or opined that IRB approval was unnecessary. Under HIPAA, however, a physician must obtain informed consent from each individual patient in order to review his or her health information and report it (even anonymously) or be able to demonstrate that it is 'not practicable' to obtain informed consent. Understandably, some IRBs interpret 'not practicable' extremely conservatively in order to protect themselves and their institutions from a stricter interpretation that might be made by federal auditors.

Adverse effects of this HIPAA provision were noted early by other writers.[2–4] Previous researchers have noted that applications for IRB approval increased, but nearly 70% of the applicants fail to complete the IRB process because of the increased documentation requirements; and there was been a drop of approximately 25% in retrospective case research.[2]

While one might argue that there are potential benefits to this situation, they certainly seem to be overshadowed by the drawbacks. The brightest 'silver lining' to this regulatory cloud is the possibility that it may stimulate more prospective controlled research, since the IRB regulatory hurdles can be nearly as imposing for a chart review as they are for a prospective invasive surgical study. Hence, one might theorize that if investigators are required to jump through most of the same hoops anyway, perhaps they might proceed with the longer, more complex evidence-based study. However, although the theory sounds good, that is not the way it works in practice, especially for medical students and residents. Rather, this regulation impedes and stifles young researchers, and it probably discourages many who might otherwise have been academically productive.

Throughout my career, I have taught medical students and residents continuously. Like many of my colleagues, I believe that scholarly activity is essential to intellectually vital medical practice, and that writing and research are habits that should be developed early. I have always provided training and support for students' and residents' scholarly activities, and even third-year medical students have been informed that some scholarly activity is expected during their rotation if they wish to receive an 'honors' grade. Until HIPAA, this encouragement led many students to start their first research projects and write their first papers, many of which were chart reviews. Moreover, many of them were scholarly and insightful, and they often led to clinical insights and additional research to improve patient care. Now, HIPAA has made such research virtually impossible unless projects are planned and IRB applications are filed months in advance of these students' rotations.

There is certainly no way that a student (even with substantial faculty help) can prepare the multiple complex forms required by an IRB, submit them, and have them reviewed, revised, resubmitted, and approved during a 3 or 4-week rotation. As a result, too many students simply give up on the idea of writing papers and do other things rather than dealing with HIPAA-imposed IRB bureaucracy.

While residents can be more productive because they have longer periods during which they can go through the process, they, too, are spending less time on retrospective reviews than they used to, and they do not appear to be compensating by doing more prospective, controlled studies. They are simply doing less research. It is almost hard to blame them. In some cases, the amount of time and writing involved in obtaining IRB approval exceeds that required for reviewing charts, collating data, and drafting a paper. This is especially true if the IRB requires that they obtain consent from each of the 50 or 100 or 200 patients whose charts they want to review.

Physicians, legislators, and hospital administrators need to work together to find solutions to this problem. While I believe that it was not an intended consequence of the HIPAA regulations, its implications for medical knowledge and academic medical practice are disturbing. Various solutions have been suggested and tried. Nationwide or institution-wide de-identified databases are helping to solve the problem, but they do not always permit study of the kind of subtleties that can be obtained from a complete medical record.

I created a consent form for participation in research on the outcomes of otolaryngology treatment that contained all the appropriate HIPAA language and presented it to each of my patients at the time of their initial visit. It required a signature and had a check box in which each patient could consent to (or decline) the anonymous use of his/her personal data for research. The IRB at my previous institution approved this form, but when I changed institutions in 2006, my new IRB rejected it as 'too general', requiring a separate consent form for each individual paper contemplated.

The HIPAA obstacles to medical research constitute a threat to medical education and good clinical care and should be addressed. Probably the best solution would be an amendment to HIPAA acknowledging that consent is unnecessary for retrospective research. Perhaps it is time for all of us to contact our legislators and get this law fixed.

References

1. Kilbridge P. The cost of HIPAA compliance. *N Engl J Med* 2003;348(15):1423–24.
2. O'Herrin JK, Fost N, Kudsk KA. Health Insurance Portability Accountability Act (HIPAA) regulations: Effect on medical record research. *Ann Surg* 2004;239(6):772–76; discussion 776–78.
3. Kulnych J, Kom D. The effect of the new federal medical-privacy rule on research. *N Engl J Med* 2002;346(3):201–4.

4. Henke PK, Fewel M, Fewel M. Surgical research and the new privacy laws. *Bull Am Coll Su* 2007;92(6):26–9.

Reprinted with modifications by permission of Vendome Group from:
    Sataloff RT. HIPAA: An impediment to research. *ENT J* 2008;87(4):182–4.

16. Evidence-based medicine

The quality and credibility of medical publications vary substantially. The greatest problem associated with publishing information that is not entirely valid is that it might mislead physicians in their clinical management of patients. This is true particularly because some published literature looks quite believable at first reading, even though it does not stand up to closer scrutiny. Recently, emphasis on evidence-based medicine (EBM) has sought to address this problem.

Increasing emphasis has been placed on improving the quality of medical literature. Many medical journals are skewing their editorial-selection process toward reporting evidence-based research classified as 'strong'. In addition, many journals are moving toward publishing evidence classification of articles, and of references cited in articles, to help the reader evaluate the information. Therefore, to better assess and improve the quality of published manuscripts, physicians should be familiar with the current standards and classification of research.

Movement toward EBM does not necessarily mean that every article published must be the result of a double-blind, placebo-controlled trial. This is fortunate for publishers, because if that were the case, we would have far fewer journals. Nevertheless, the growing awareness of the importance of EBM emphasizes the need for critical analysis and scrutiny of every article we read. It also provides a structure to help evaluate the credibility of a publication. Hence, it is valuable for all physicians to acquire a basic understanding of EBM.

In order to approach a problem using the EBM paradigm, the information sought on a typical topic is structured into questions that can be answered. These questions should be addressed efficiently, using the best possible evidence (see information below on levels of evidence) to elucidate the answers. The evidence obtained is evaluated critically to determine its validity and to determine whether it answers the questions in a useful way. The results are then combined with information based upon clinical expertise and previous experience gleaned from the literature. Then, outcomes are evaluated. This systematic approach to expanding scientific knowledge is the essence of the EBM 'movement', although a great deal of attention is paid to one portion of this paradigm, specifically: the level of evidence (LOE).

The LOE is supposed to help a reader understand the credibility of the results presented. Are they valid? That is, are they unbiased and true? Validity does not necessarily predict clinical relevance, but it is certainly important to understand whether reported information is believable before deciding whether to rely upon it for changes in clinical management.

Evidence may be classified into four categories. However, the reader should be aware that numerous other classification schemes exist and grade evidence into five or more categories. Level I evidence (the highest category) includes randomized, controlled trials; meta-analyses; systematic reviews; and reports of diagnostic sensitivity and specificity. In randomized, controlled trials, two identical groups are divided randomly into a control group and an experimental group; and both groups are followed prospectively for specific endpoints often using a 'gold standard' for case definition. Meta-analyses involve quantitative synthesis (or pooling) of data from numerous independent clinical trials. Readers should be aware that while metanalyses are classified as Level I evidence, they are intrinsically limited by the quality of the studies they include. Systematic reviews utilize specific methods to identify primary studies, assess their quality, and review research their data. Diagnostic sensitivity and specificity studies report the true positive and negative rates for diagnostic tests.

Level II evidence may be provided through a prospective study that includes a narrower spectrum of subjects with the suspected condition, or through a well-designed retrospective study including a broad spectrum of subjects with a condition established by a 'gold standard.' These subjects are compared with a broad spectrum of controls, with the test that is being evaluated applied in a blinded fashion. Cohort studies are classified as Level II evidence. They involve groups of people who are identified because of their exposure to a particular agent, for example, and who are followed for selected outcomes. In Level III studies, evidence is acquired retrospectively, either using a narrow spectrum of subjects who have the established condition or retrospective controls, but in which the test or topic under investigation is still applied in a blinded fashion. Case control studies (Level III evidence) compare subjects who have a specific condition with matched 'controls', retrospectively analyzing differences between the groups. Level IV includes any study design in which the test under investigation is not applied in a blinded evaluation, or in which evidence is provided by descriptive case series without controls. Cross-sectional surveys (surveys or interviews of a subject population) and case reports or short case series are examples of Level IV evidence. Expert opinion, in the form of opinion from a preeminent authority or consensus from a group of authorities, also constitutes Level IV evidence. Anecdote and conversation are not classified with a defined evidence level.

It should be obvious immediately that lower rank does not necessarily mean invalid or 'bad' information. In fact, well-synthesized expert opinion from a panel of world leaders may provide invaluable information, as may well-written case reports or especially case series. Nevertheless, it is important for readers of medical literature to recognize that the validity of conclusions drawn from Level III or Level II studies (or lower level reports) might not be as certain as the validity of conclusions derived from Level I studies. Skepticism is wise when interpreting any medical literature, and physicians should be cautious about what to believe.

The old adage 'Save me from the doctor who has just read a paper' calls to mind the pitfalls associated with less-than-critical absorption of information from the medical literature. Evaluating each paper for LOE helps physicians sort out articles on which they should rely from those with insufficient power to support a clinical decision.

In addition to using LOE to evaluate published literature, otolaryngologists should also remember classification of evidence when designing a study or preparing to write a paper. Often, it takes surprisingly little extra effort to increase the credibility of a study by modifying the design to increase its evidence level. This can sometimes make the difference between valid and invalid results, and between acceptance and rejection of a manuscript.

Medical writers and publishers are still struggling with sensible adoption of the principles of EBM. Overall, the trend toward a more rigorous study design appears healthy, and heightened awareness of the strengths and weaknesses of the study design of each published paper is certainly advantageous to physicians and our patients.

Reprinted with modifications by permission of Vendome Group from:
    Sataloff RT. Evidence-based medicine. *ENT J* 2006;85(10):624–5.
    Sataloff RT. Evidence-based research. *ENT J* 2004;83(9):599.

17. Evidence-based medicine: Yet more concerns

This author has expressed reservations previously about the rush to evidence-based medicine (EBM).[1] I have continued to follow writings on this topic with interest over the years, and my concerns about the strong emphasis on evidence-based research and the implication that it results in superior validity have not diminished. I am comforted to know I am not alone. Many authors have expressed skepticism, some in articles well worth reviewing. One example was a commentary published in 2016, 'Evidence-based medicine has been hijacked: A report to David Sackett' by Dr. John Ioannidis.[2] This article might have been missed by physicians who do not follow the *Journal of Clinical Epidemiology*. It was sent to me by my colleague Dr. Brian McKinnon. The article is both entertaining and insightful.

Dr. Ioannidis is an epidemiologist and professor of medicine with appointments in three departments and a Meta-research Innovation Center at Stanford University, who has studied EBM for more than a decade, and whose insights might be different (and potentially more sophisticated) than those of many doctors (certainly including this author). I will not recount his observations in detail in this chapter (as tempting as that is), because I would prefer to encourage readers to review them for themselves. However, this chapter summarizes some of the highlights that I find credible, predictable, and somewhat disturbing.

Previously, I have noted that EBM has some intrinsic drawbacks and limitations, and that prospective, double-blind research is not the only literature worth publishing. Moreover, the fact that a study appears to meet the criteria for high-quality, evidence-based research does not necessarily mean that its conclusions are valid. Nevertheless, EBM may have a greater likelihood of producing valid (or at least defensible) results than other, less rigorous research designs, and it has developed a certain cache. Hence, we should not be surprised with the argument put forth by Dr Ioannidis that EBM has been 'hijacked'.

Ioannidis is correct in noting that as EBM has become more influential, the temptation to exploit it for commercial purposes has grown. A large number of randomized trials are sponsored by, or actually done by, industries affected commercially by the results of the research. We used to joke (sort of) that a good statistician could prove anything. Good statisticians are intrinsic to EBM, and results can be biased by subtleties of study design and data analysis that might not be obvious to readers.

In my opinion, this might be particularly dangerous because there is a growing tendency for readers to believe that if an article meets the highest standards of evidence-based research, then it has been vetted already, and its conclusions can be believed. Therefore, readers might be tempted to read highly rated EBM articles less critically and less incisively than articles that do not have the imprimatur of EBM (I have no evidence to support this suspicion, of course, and it is not part of the wisdom put forth by Ioannidis).

Along with other EBM, Ioannidis attacks meta-analyses and guidelines as having 'become a factory' and also, as largely serving 'vested interests'. I agree with his observations that a great deal of funds (private and federal) are expended on projects, including some meta-analyses, that have little relevance to clinical medicine, especially to improving outcomes.

I would add that all of us should remember that meta-analyses combine data from numerous published studies. While this statistical technique can be valuable in detecting trends and extracting information missed because of smaller numbers in each component study, it does not correct fundamental design flaws and other errors in the studies that it includes. In fact, the technique can compound them. Worse, the fact that a publication is a 'meta-analysis' might give it credibility similar to that of other EBM in the eyes of many readers who might believe conclusions that are supported statistically by the meta-analyses, but that are not correct.

All of our journals strive for quality, and EBM has become synonymous with quality in the eyes of many academicians, readers and even some editors. All of us need to remain vigilant and to recognize that there is no approach to research that ensures truth in and of itself and that, like the results of all other investigations, products of EBM are subject to unintentional, or even intentional, bias. We still need to read with a critical eye.

References

1. Sataloff RT. Evidence-based medicine. *ENT J* 2006;85(10):624–5.
2. Ioannidis JPA. Evidence-based medicine has been hijacked: A report to David Sackett. *J Clin Epidemiol* 2016;73:82–6.

Reprinted with modifications by permission of Vendome Group from:
   Sataloff RT. Evidence-based medicine: Yet more concerns. *ENT J* 2017;96(7):234.

18. Clinical trials: The case for registration

A clinical trial is any research project that assigns human subjects prospectively to comparison groups and compares the relationships between a medical intervention and a health outcome. The CONSORT (Consolidated Standards of Reporting Trials) guidelines were established to assist investigators in achieving high-quality research design and reporting[1] but, unfortunately, many clinical trials remain unpublished.

Some researchers fail to publish because of negative or inconclusive outcomes; other investigators have given up control, and a funding organization has refused publication. Failure to disseminate clinical trial information (regardless of outcome) has caused considerable concern within the scientific community, particularly among editors of medical journals.[2]

This problem is both ethical and practical. By definition, clinical trials involve patient volunteers. In many cases, patients have accepted considerable inconvenience, discomfort, and risk in choosing to participate in clinical studies. Often, they are aware that they will receive no personal benefit from the study, but they have volunteered to assist medical science in helping future patients. Clinical trial volunteers have a right to know the outcomes of the studies in which they have participated. In addition, we should be able to assure them that physicians will have access to whatever information the study has generated, regardless of its conclusions.

The International Committee of Medical Journal Editors has issued a statement including the opinion that every clinical trial should be registered in a complete public database in order for an article about that trial to be accepted for review by a medical journal.[2] I believe this opinion is correct and should be endorsed by all medical journals.

Trial registries are readily accessible on the Internet.[3] For example, the website ClinicalTrials.gov makes such information available for both physicians and patients. Registration of Phase I trials (pharmacokinetics or drug toxicity) and Phase II (dosing) trials is recommended, but Phase III trial registration should be mandatory. Phase III trials are designed to help determine clinical practice. Evidence from every such project is potentially valuable. Even equivocal or negative results provide the scientific community with important information about what not to do, as well as what not to spend time or money researching again (at least using the same experimental design).

Registering a clinical trial on the ClinicalTrials.gov website is easy. Investigators must first apply for a Protocol Registration System (PRS) account. There are two types: organization and individual PRS accounts. Organization accounts generally have multiple users and are intended to register all the trials being conducted at an organization, with individual accounts used to register trials conducted by a single investigator.[4] Within two business days, ClinicalTrials.gov will create the account and send an e-mail with instructions on how to log in to the PRS, in order to register a trial.

Ethical conduct of clinical research does not end with Institutional Review Board approval and entry of patients; investigators have an obligation to their subjects and the medical community to disseminate study findings. Registration should be expected for all clinical studies that started enrolling patients after September 2005, and registration should be required before such studies are reviewed for publication.

References

1. Moher D, Schulz KE, Altman DE. CONSORT Group. The Consort statement: Revised recommendations for improving the quality of reports of parallel-group randomized trials. *Ann Intern Med* 2001;134:657–62.
2. DeAngelis CD, Drazen JM, Frizelle FA, et al. Clinical trial registration: A statement from the International Committee of Medical Journal Editors. *JAMA* 2004;292:1363–4.
3. Haug C, Gotzsche PC, Schroeder TV. Registries and registration of clinical trials. *N Engl J Med* 2005;353:2811–12.
4. U.S. National Library of Medicine. 'How to apply for an account'. U.S. National Institutes of Health, Department of Health and Human Services. http://prsinfo.

clinicaltrials.gov/gettingOrgAccount.html. Accessed September 19, 2018.

Reprinted with modifications by permission of Vendome Group from:
Sataloff RT. Clinical trials: The case for registration. *ENT J* 2006;85(6):352–3.

19. Drug development research: The process

Physicians often are involved in clinical trials, and nearly all of us read publications based on pharmaceutical research. However, many physicians who are not involved routinely in drug development may be unfamiliar with the stages in the drug development process, and with related terminology. Understanding such information helps interpret literature.

Briefly, there are several stages in the drug development process. The first stages are preclinical. Once an idea has been put forth for a new product (the creation of new product concepts will not be addressed in this chapter), the investigator and/or sponsor initiates research by testing the new product in vitro. In vitro studies are followed by animal studies designed to provide information about toxic effects and the pharmacologic nature and behavior of the investigational drug. Following successful preclinical research, clinical research may be initiated.

The first step in clinical research is to apply to the U.S. Food and Drug Administration (FDA) for an Investigational New Drug (IND) application. This is a complex application. Before issuing an IND number, the FDA reviews all preclinical research data, scientific information on the formulation of the investigational drug, manufacturing procedures and expertise, the qualifications of the proposed investigator, and the proposed clinical protocol. An IND is required not only for investigational drugs proposed by pharmaceutical companies or other private entities, but even for those proposed by federal agencies or the National Institutes of Health (NIH) intramural programs, prior to human use.

Phase I trials involve a small number of subjects, usually between 10 and 100. These trials may include patients or normal volunteers. If the drug involves substantial risk or is likely to cause harm (such as immunosuppressive therapy or cytotoxic chemotherapy), it still is appropriate to use patients so long as they are fully informed and give their consent. Typically, unless the drug is targeted specifically for women's health concerns, Phase I trials seek normal male volunteers to assess the investigational drug's initial exposure to an entire population.

Phase I trials reveal information about pharmacologic action, metabolism, and toxicity in humans and help create a preliminary, dose-related profile of side effects.

Phase II trials are tightly controlled studies with strict inclusion and exclusion criteria. They include a larger but still a relatively small number of subjects, usually not exceeding several hundred. Phase II trials evaluate the effectiveness of the drug in treating a particular condition in patients, and they provide further information about short-term side effects and risks.

Phase III trials may include thousands of patients. Generally, these trials are designed for rapid recruitment of subjects and are approved only after data from Phase II trials indicate that the drug is effective for the condition under study. Phase III trials provide greater insight into safety and efficacy, as well as risks, effects, and side effects. The risks/benefits information developed from Phase III trials affect FDA-approved labeling of the drug when it is brought to market.

An investigational drug can be brought to market if Phase III studies indicate adequate safety and efficacy. In order to obtain permission to market a new pharmaceutical product, a New Drug Application (NDA) is required. This is also a complex and exhaustive application that includes all clinical data, all safety data from clinical studies, drug formulation and manufacturing information, and the results of at least two substantive Phase III trials.

Phase IV trials may be conducted by a pharmaceutical company after a product is available on the market and has received FDA approval. Phase IV trials are prudent and informative, but they typically are not required by the FDA. A company or investigator may choose to perform Phase IV studies to investigate the effects of different doses or dosing schedules from those used in Phase II and Phase III trials; to determine the behavior of the drug in different patient populations or in patients with earlier or more advanced stages of disease; to monitor long-term effectiveness of the new agent; to compare the drug with other drugs available on the market; or to compare the cost effectiveness of the drug with that of other products.

There is an analogous, similarly rigorous process required for development of devices that has been required by the FDA since 1980. That process will not be discussed in detail in this chapter, but it is important to recognize that devices also must undergo clinical trials before they can be brought to market. The rigor and expense of the clinical trials process varies depending upon whether the device is determined to be a 'significant risk device' or 'non-significant risk device'. Physicians should be aware that such regulations exist and may influence greatly the viability of creative new device concepts (including surgical instruments and, particularly, implants) because the costs associated with federal approval can be prohibitive.

Physicians interested in more information on device development often can obtain it most easily through their institutional review boards.

Drug (and device) development is complex, and it is regulated strictly to ensure public safety. Requirements affect the timing of development, product availability, product cost, and other factors. Since physicians evaluate new products routinely on behalf of our patients, and since we read so much literature arising from new product development and testing, it is important for us to be cognizant of the requirements and stages of product development and to understand the various phases of the process. Such information is invaluable in interpreting the massive quantities of new information to which we are exposed daily.

Reprinted with modifications by permission of Vendome Group from:
Sataloff RT. Drug development research: The process. *ENT J* 2008;87(8):420–2.

20. Understanding the regulation of pharmaceutical drug promotion

Natalie A. Krane, M.D.
Department of Otolaryngology–Head and Neck Surgery, Oregon Health & Science University, Portland, Oregon

Robert T. Sataloff, M.D., D.M.A., F.A.C.S.
Professor and Chairman, Department of Otolaryngology–Head and Neck Surgery, Senior Associate Dean for Clinical Academic Specialties, Drexel University College of Medicine

Yearly, billions of dollars are funneled into the promotion of pharmaceutical drugs to healthcare professionals (HCPs) and consumers. In 2012, roughly 27 billion U.S. dollars were spent on promotional activity by the pharmaceutical industry, with more than 24 billion dollars spent on marketing to physicians.[1] Promotional print items, speaker series, direct-to-consumer advertising (DTCA), detail aids (promotional material left behind by sales reps for physician perusal), and the like are regulated heavily, and it is known that pharmaceutical marketing via DTCA affects both consumer and HCP behavior.[2] However, the details of such regulation are not common knowledge, even though pharmaceutical promotion infiltrates daily medical practice and life. Physicians should be familiar with regulations, the risks associated with pharmaceutical promotion, and opportunities to help ensure dissemination of accurate information.

The established practice at most pharmaceutical companies, although it is different at each organization, has the same goal: to ensure each promotional item developed by marketing teams is in congruence with the U.S. Food and Drug Administration's Office of Prescription Drug Promotion (FDA OPDP) regulations and guidance documents. The team implemented at each company that reviews and critiques promotional materials consists of marketing, legal and regulatory representation, in addition to two medical liaisons, one of whom is responsible for ensuring the accuracy of the medical facts presented (reference and statistical review), and a medical doctor whose primary focus is on the accuracy, applicability and medical relevance of the promotional material. The gold standard by which all promotional material is judged is the package insert (PI), which is an FDA-approved document containing indications for use, dosing and administration, safety and risk information, approval study data, and much more.

The OPDP regulations and guidance documents provide a framework within which the pharmaceutical industry can develop commercial material containing claims that are accurate, balanced, and based on the PI ('on-label') indications. However, this framework is not always black and white. The gray area spreads widely, allowing for differences in interpretation and implementation. When this framework is breached, the OPDP can distribute an 'Untitled Letter' instructing the company to which it was sent to cease promotion of the offending material immediately for the reasons outlined within the letter.

More egregious offenses result in a 'Warning Letter' instructing companies not only to cease promotion, but also to 'right their wrong', which commonly involves releasing an advertisement containing corrections (a costly endeavor) and/or distributing a 'Dear Healthcare Professional' letter.

Both Untitled and Warning letters are available to the public on the FDA's website and are used frequently by pharmaceutical companies to learn from others' errors. They also can be beneficial to HCPs by bringing to light the common issues involved with pharmaceutical promotion. The most common citations issued in Untitled or Warning Letters are for promotional endeavors containing claims that overstate efficacy, including unsubstantiated efficacy claims, or portray superiority; promotional items that are misleading because of inaccuracies and/or ambiguity; and materials that contain omissions and/or minimize safety and risk information.

Other common citations address broadening the indication for which the drug is approved or broadening the patient population for which the drug is approved, and inclusion of quality-of-life claims that are often hard to prove with substantial evidence. Promotional materials often are brought under fire for an unbalanced presentation of efficacy and safety information. Essentially, the emphasis on a drug's efficacy outweighs the important safety information, which should be distributed evenly throughout the promotional material or presentation in question.

Pharmaceutical companies are obligated to submit their promotional materials to the FDA's OPDP at the time of promotional distribution, thereby allowing promotional material to circulate and/or be presented for a long while prior to a possible citation by the OPDP. It should be noted, however, that even though submission of promotional materials is required at the time of first use, the FDA does not, in fact, review all distributed promotional materials. This remains an important reason for HCPs to be vigilant regarding pharmaceutical marketing.

There is also an option for industry to submit promotional material for preapproval, before the first use, which may be the route taken for DTCA or new website material, for example. For these materials, a breach of regulation can result in a hefty financial loss for the company because of the required remediation expenditure. The preapproval process involves review by the OPDP and provides an opportunity to receive feedback prior to the distribution of promotional material. However, this process does not guarantee that the final promotional material will be in accordance with regulations.

Social media platforms also are used by the pharmaceutical industry. This avenue of promotion is relatively new. Being so, clear guidance surrounding the development of promotional material distributed by social media does not exist and releasing material in this way involves 'trial and error', at best. Applying print regulations to social media promotional material is exceedingly difficult, as multiple elements, such as communication on social media (e.g., consumer commentary), are not contained within print promotion. Therefore, developing social media promotional material imposes a substantially increased risk, resulting in a sector of promotion that might not be fully compliant with the OPDP recommendations.

In addition, the use of technology such as tablets by sales representatives, instead of print material, is increasing. Originally, it was believed there would be less control over the way the material was presented, and that advancements such as the ability to zoom in on certain portions of the material might leave important safety information minimized and the overall impression unbalanced. However, it was realized that there actually is an ability to obtain more control over what the sales representatives promote. For example, a detail or sales aid can be programmed to display fair balance safety 'pop-ups' for a predetermined amount of time, something that a print sales aid cannot offer.

The FDA's 'Bad Ad' program is a campaign that includes HCPs in the regulation of promotional activity by the pharmaceutical industry. It is a means by which questionable promotional activity can be reported directly to the FDA for review and, if necessary, for citation. With the continuing technologic advancements and increasing means by which the pharmaceutical industry can promote, HCPs can be increasingly effective in governing pharmaceutical promotion. Physicians should remain critical in their reading of pharmaceutical materials, vigilant in their search for misleading information to avoid practice errors that might affect patient care adversely, and proactive in participating in federal efforts to ensure accurate and balanced promotion of pharmaceutical products.

References

1. Cegedim Strategic Data. 2012 U.S. Pharmaceutical Company Promotion Spending. Updated January 2013. www.skainfo.com/health_care_market_reports/2012_promotional_spending.pdf. Accessed August 13, 2018.
2. Kravitz RL, Epstein RM, Feldman MD, et al. Influence of patients' requests for direct-to-consumer advertised antidepressants: A randomized controlled trial. *JAMA* 2005;293(16):1995–2002.

Reprinted with modifications by permission of Vendome Group from:
Krane NA, Sataloff RT. Understanding the regulation of pharmaceutical drug promotion. *ENT J* 2014;93(12):486–8.

21. Quality of reporting in randomized trials

A great deal of emphasis has been placed recently on the importance of high-quality evidence in medical literature. Placebo-controlled, randomized, prospective studies are valued especially highly. However, the fact that a study is placebo-controlled, randomized, and prospective does not necessarily mean that it was well designed and well-reported, or that the conclusions are valid. For example, Sinha et al. highlighted this important issue in a review of randomized trials published in high-quality surgical journals.[1] The quality of the journal was determined by its impact factor.

In analyzing the literature, Sinha et al. used the Consolidated Standards of Reporting Trials (CONSORT) statement published in the *Journal of the American Medical Association* (JAMA) in 1996.[2] The CONSORT statement resulted from international collaboration among biomedical editors, clinicians, and statisticians. In order to correct shortcomings in reporting of trial methodology, they promulgated a standardized framework to assist authors in reporting findings of clinical trials completely and transparently. The CONSORT statement was revised in 2001,[3] and it can be accessed at http://www.consort-statement.org/. Although following CONSORT guidelines improves reporting of clinical trials, and although the statement is accepted by many biomedical journals, it has not been used as widely as one might wish.

In their study, Sinha et al. analyzed 42 randomized, controlled trials (RCTs), calculating their Jadad[4] scores. The Jadad score is determined through assessment of questions addressing randomization, blinding, and reporting of withdrawals and dropouts from studies.[4] The Jadad score has been validated as a scale for assessing trial reporting quality and is used to distinguish low-quality from high-quality studies. Sinha et al. used a Jadad score of ≥3 for their threshold (a conservative choice, since some authors require a score of ≥4). In the three high-quality journals that they evaluated, only 40% of 42 RCTs achieved a Jadad score of >3. Only 32.5% of the RCTs reported methodology adequately, and only 17% provided adequate reporting of adverse events.

Such self-analysis in the general surgical literature is commendable. In most specialties, we rely upon published literature to guide our patient care decisions (among other things). When we read reports that are given the highest evidence ratings, and when we see that they are prospective, randomized trials, many of us are inclined to believe the results. However, it seems appropriate for us to critique these publications as rigorously as possible, both in terms of design and in terms of quality and completeness of reporting.

All of us should be aware of the CONSORT statement. Although I have not followed Sinha's example and performed a similar analysis on otolaryngology literature yet, I believe this should be done. Only through constant, rigorous assessment of the quality of our published data can we hope to arrive at true information that can be applied ethically, and with confidence, to the care of our patients. Journals in every field should consider adopting the CONSORT statement and educating reviewers to consider it (and the Jadad score) when evaluating randomized trials submitted for publication.

References

1. Sinha S, Sinha S, Ashby E, et al. Quality of reporting in randomized trials published in high-quality surgical journals. *J Am Coll Surg* 2009;209(5):565–71.
2. Begg C, Cho M, Eastwood S, et al. Improving the quality of reporting of randomized controlled trials. The CONSORT statement. *JAMA* 1996;27(8):637–39.
3. Moher D, Schulz KF, Altman DG. CONSORT GROUP (Consolidated Standards of Reporting Trials). The CONSORT statement: Revised recommendations for improving the quality of reports of parallel-group randomized trials. *Ann Intern Med* 2001;134(8):657–62.
4. Jadad AR, Moore RA, Carroll D, et al. Assessing the quality of reports of randomized clinical trials: Is blinding necessary? *Controlled Clin Trials* 1996;17(1):1–12.

Reprinted with modifications by permission from Vendome Group from:
  Sataloff RT. Quality of reporting in randomized trials. *ENT J* 2010;89(4):50.

22. Human subject research or quality improvement project?

Most physicians are learning to adapt to quality-based reimbursement. It might be helpful to remember that the initiative to define and improve quality is nearly two decades old and is ongoing. Seminal publications from the Institute of Medicine in 2000 described the problems and potential solutions,[1-2] and more recent publications document continued efforts at quality improvement.[3] Quality measures have been implemented by not only the American College of Surgeons through the American College of Surgeons National Quality Improvement Program (ACS NSQIP),[4] but also by the Centers for Medicare and Medicaid Services (CMS) through its Surgical Care Improvement Project (SCIP).[5] Surgical specialists need to be involved in quality improvement projects (QIP) in order to help determine appropriate quality definitions and measures for each specialty. However, the differences between quality improvement projects and human subjects research (HSR) requiring institutional review board (IRB) approval are not always clear. This subject was reviewed by Raval et al in 2014,[6] and areas of confusion and controversy have not been clarified much in the intervening years.

Research is 'a systematic investigation, including research development, testing and evaluation, designed to develop or contribute to generalizable knowledge', as defined by the Federal Code of Regulations (32 CFR 219.102 [D]).[7] Research is designed to clarify and expand understanding of a specific disease, problem or treatment, and to add to the profession's fund of knowledge. Quality improvement projects are not designed to expand generalizable knowledge. Rather, they are used to determine whether an accepted behavior or practice is being utilized locally and if not, to seek to change the behavior of healthcare providers to bring their actions into compliance with accepted norms.

Raval et al summarized the effects of QIP as including interventions (including physical procedures such as venipuncture or biopsies) through which data are gathered; manipulation of a subject or environment for quality improvement (QI) research purposes; communication or interpersonal contact between the researcher and subject; and acquisition of personal health information that is not made public, but which is available to the investigator. In general, QIPs do not include control groups. QIPs generally do not involve assembling a data set that has been built and then had the subjects de-identified. However, most QIPs are, or come close to being, HSR.

HSR is well-known to most of physicians. It is performed for the purpose of enhancing knowledge in the field generally, and acquiring information that will expand our understanding of diseases, and/or alter evaluation and treatment. It requires IRB approval, and subjects must be de-identified. An IRB might determine that formal IRB application and approval, and informed consent, can be waived if the research does not adversely affect the rights and welfare of the subjects, poses no more than minimal risk, could not be performed if consent were required, and meets other specific criteria. For research, the Health Insurance Portability and Accountability Act (HIPAA) requires de-identification of personal health information for subjects to be used in research. There are two methods of de-identifying data. Specific information can be deleted from data sets (the safe-harbor method). Alternatively, personal identifiers can be removed from each subject, to the point at which the data cannot be traced back to individual subjects. There are national data sets available that have been de-identified. For example, de-identified Medicare billing data are available. So is information from the Agency for Health Care Research and Quality's Healthcare Cost and Utilization Project, the ACS NSQIP participant use file. The SEER database also is de-identified. So, a study using these databases typically does not require formal IRB review and approval. However, in most cases it is appropriate to submit the proposed research to an IRB in order to have a formal determination and letter stating that the project has been evaluated and found to be exempt.

While it is important for us to perform quality improvement projects as well as human research, it is essential that we take all necessary precautions to avoid violating the rights of patients, the laws governing human subject research, and the ethics of such investigations (summarized briefly by Raval et al[6]). Nevertheless, physicians must be involved. If we do not perform quality improvement projects and the appropriate research within our specialty and define what should be measured and what constitutes 'quality,' someone else will do it for us; and that is not likely to result in valid, reliable or practical measures. Interested physicians should proceed enthusiastically, but knowledgably. Consultation with a senior representative of the institutional review board, and with a statistician, prior to beginning research is invaluable.

References

1. Kohn LT, Corrigan JM, Donaldson MS (eds). To Err Is Human: Building A Safer Health System. Committee on Quality of Health Care in America, Institute of Medicine. Washington, DC: National Academy Press; 2000.
2. Institute of Medicine. Crossing the Quality Chasm: A New Health System for the 21st Century. Washington, DC: National Academy Press; 2001.
3. U.S. Department of Health and Human Services. National Quality Strategy. 2011 Report to Congress: National Strategy for Quality Improvement in Health Care. March 2011. http://www.ahrq.gov/workingforquality/nqs/nqs2011annlrpt.htm. Accessed August 13, 2018.
4. American College of Surgeons National Surgical Quality Improvement Program. About ACS NSQIP. http://site.acsnsqip.org/about. Accessed August 13, 2018.
5. The Joint Commission. Specifications Manual for Joint Commission National Quality Core Measures (Version 2010B). Surgical Care Improvement Project. Set measures. March 2011. https://manual.jointcommission.org/releases/archive/TJC2010B1/SurgicalCareImprovementProject.html. Accessed August 13, 2018.
6. Raval MV, Sakran JV, Medbery RL, et al. Distinguishing QI projects from human subjects research: Ethical and practical considerations. *Bulletin ACS* 2014;99(7):21–7.
7. U.S. Department of Health and Human Services. Code of Federal Regulations: Title 45: Public Welfare, Part 46: Protection of Human Subjects. Last revised January 15, 2009. http://www.hhs.gov/ohrp/humansubjects/guidance/45cfr46.html. Accessed August 13, 2018.

Reprinted with modifications by permission from Vendome Group from:
Sataloff RT. Human Subject Research or Quality Improvement Project? *ENT J*, in press.

23. Practice parameters and clinical practice guidelines: Science, politics, and problems

Physicians in various specialties have not been equally prolific in promulgating practice parameters and technology assessments. Many fields have more clinical practice guidelines than practice parameters, but even many of these were developed through a relatively informal process until recently. Since neither practice parameters (or technology assessments) nor clinical practice guidelines have been a major focus for many physicians, many of us are unfamiliar with all their potential values, or the problems that may be associated with them.

Clinical practice guidelines should be distinguished from practice parameters. Virtually all specialties have at least some clinical practice guidelines. They are essentially consensus statements on a specific topic and are intended 'to assist practitioner and patient decisions about appropriate healthcare for specific clinical circumstances'.[1] While the development process usually includes a review of literature and evidence, guidelines typically contain opinion (it might just be the consensus of the guidelines committee that developed them) that is not always supported entirely by irrefutable evidence.

For example, the American Academy of Otolaryngology–Head and Neck Surgery has issued such guidelines and policies. They often are developed by Academy committees and are published to document our best recommendations regarding management of clinical conditions. The opinions developed by such committees go through a rigorous review process and are vetted by the board before being adopted by the Academy. They form a synthesis of the judgments of many of our best subspecialists and have been valuable to our membership. So far, they have not resulted in significant legal action, but not all medical organizations have been that fortunate.

For example, the Infectious Diseases Society of America (IDSA) issued updated clinical practice guidelines for the diagnosis and treatment of Lyme disease in 2006.[2] The subsequent problems faced by the IDSA were reviewed in an enlightening article in the Journal of the American Medical Association (JAMA).[3] Shortly after the guidelines were issued, the Connecticut attorney general alleged that IDSA had violated state antitrust law by advising against long-term antibiotics to treat 'chronic Lyme disease (CLD)'. The IDSA, the Centers for Disease Control and Prevention, and the National Institutes of Health agree with that recommendation and that 'despite extensive study, no clear evidence has emerged to support the contention that CLD results from a past or persistent Lyme disease infection'.[3]

Despite the scientific basis for the IDSA guidelines, protest by a CLD advocacy group led the Connecticut attorney general to launch an investigation of IDSA's guideline writing process. IDSA spent more than a quarter of a million dollars in legal expenses before settling with the attorney general and agreeing to a review panel to reassess the 2006 guidelines and processes.[4] If the process for developing clinical guidelines is not rigorous, if there is any potential conflict of interest that could bias members of the committee and if there is not transparency, clinical guidelines can open individuals and organizations not only to civil suits, but also to antitrust litigation. While clinical guidelines are important and serve a valuable function, it appears to be time for physicians to look more closely at our processes.

In contrast to clinical guidelines, practice parameters and technology assessments do not contain non-evidence-based consensus opinion. Rather, they synthesize all published evidence regarding a specific topic and follow a rigorous development process. I have been involved with this process, and its purity is monitored carefully. The American Academy of Neurology (AAN) was probably the most active organization early in development of practice parameters, having published more than 100 practice parameters and technology assessments between the mid 1990s and the mid-2000s.[5]

Practice parameters and technology assessments ensure transparency by publishing all aspects of the process, including search terms, strategies, databases utilized, and any other relevant information. This allows readers to judge the validity of the process. The practice-parameter committees gather evidence-based studies on the topic in question, primarily clinical studies. Each article is classified (Level I through Level IV) on the basis of strength of evidence (and risk of bias), using published criteria.[6] Members of the practice-parameter and technology-assessment committees of the AAN (who will be authors of the published practice parameters) are selected to minimize bias and ensure balance within the committee. The AAN provides oversight, and the product of the committee is expected to synthesize what is known about the topic, and to state the degree of certainty with which facts are known. Practice parameters now exist in virtually all specialties and are formulated through a similar process

The practice parameters include recommendations determined strictly from evidence-based data. The recommendations may be (A) established as effective, ineffective, or harmful; (B) probably effective, ineffective, or harmful; (C) possibly effective, ineffective, or harmful; or (U) data inadequate or conflicting; given current knowledge, treatment (test, predictor) is unproven.

Practice parameters and technology assessments have great value. They establish what is known and not known through evidence-based research. This process not only validates various treatments or tests, but it also highlights research that needs to be performed. In addition, it shines a bright light on the weaknesses in our literature. For example, in writing a practice parameter for laryngeal electromyography, we reviewed 584 articles. Only 33 qualified for inclusion on the basis of their study designs. None of the articles was Level I or Level II. Only two were Level III, and the rest were Level IV (the lowest level of evidence).[7-9] If slightly more thought had been given to study design, many of the papers reviewed could have been more credible.

Practice parameters and technology assessments also pose potential problems. For one, most physicians do not understand what they are, and they use them as clinical practice guidelines. They are not. They represent a synthesis of evidence-based data, not a consensus of expert opinion on clinical management. Furthermore, by design they are limited to addressing a specific, usually narrow, question; and it is often inappropriate to try to generalize their conclusions into the complex arena of patient management.

In this era of overwhelming information, practice parameters and technology assessments that synthesize evidence-based data, and clinical practice guidelines that combine evidence with a consensus of expert opinion, are both invaluable resources to clinicians and clinician researchers. It may be appropriate for all physicians to consider increasing our activity in these areas; but it is incumbent for us to do so with thorough appreciation for the complexities of the processes so that we can produce the best possible documents, with the least possible risk of clinical misuse or legal attack.

References

1. National Heart Lung, and Blood Institute, National Institutes of Health. About systemic evidence reviews and clinical practice guidelines. U.S. Department of Health & Human Services. https://www.nhlbi.nih.gov/node/80397. Accessed September 19, 2018.
2. Wormser GP, Dattwyler RJ, Shapiro ED, et al. The clinical assessment, treatment, and prevention of lyme disease, human granulocytic anaplasmosis, and babesiosis: Clinical practice guidelines by the Infectious Diseases Society of America. *Clin Infect Dis* 2006;43(9):1089–134.
3. Kraemer JD, Gostin LO. Science, politics, and values: The politicization of professional practice guidelines. *JAMA* 2009;301(6):665–7.
4. Klein JO. Danger ahead: Politics intrude in Infectious Diseases Society of America guideline for Lyme disease. *Clin Infect Dis* 2008;47(9):1197–9.
5. Gronseth G, French J. Practice parameters and technology assessments: What they are, what they are not, and why you should care. *Neurology* 2008;71(20):1639–43.
6. Sataloff RT. Evidence-based medicine. *ENT J* 2006;85(10): 624–5.
7. Sataloff RT, Mandel S, Ludlow C; AAEM Laryngeal Task Force. Laryngeal electromyography: An evidence-based review. *Muscle Nerve* 2003;28(6):767–72.
8. Sataloff RT, Mandel S, Mann EA, Ludlow CL. Practice parameter: Laryngeal electromyography (an evidenced-based review). *J Voice* 2004;18(2):261–74.
9. Sataloff RT, Mandel S, Mann EA, Ludlow CL. Practice parameter: Laryngeal electromyography (an evidenced-based review). *Otolaryngol HNS* 2004;130(6):770–9.

Reprinted with modifications by permission of Vendome Group from:
Sataloff RT. Practice parameters and clinical practice guidelines: Science, politics, and problems. *ENT J* 2009;88(6):946–9.

24. Centralized Otolaryngology Research Efforts (CORE) grants

Obtaining extramural funding has always been a challenge, even for full-time researchers, but perhaps especially for practicing physicians and young investigators. Among the many challenges, deciding where to submit a grant proposal can be particularly daunting.

In 1985, the American Academy of Otolaryngology-Head and Neck Surgery, now the American Academy of Otolaryngology-Head and Neck Surgery Foundation (AAO-HNSF), provided help by establishing the Centralized Otolaryngology Research Efforts (CORE) grants program.[1,2] Many (but not all) otolaryngology societies and some corporate foundations that provide research funds participate in the program, which helps unify the research application process for the specialty and assists funders and applicants by providing an expert review process. This initiative has worked well and is potentially a valuable model for other specialties.

CORE study section reviews are transmitted as recommendations to an appropriate society or other funding organization, and the funding organizations retain the ability to act on grant applications independently. The CORE program is intended to make the application process easier, help prepare young investigators for more complex funding applications (such as those for the National Institutes of

Health [NIH]), and to encourage young investigators and physicians in or out of academic centers to participate in research that will help improve our specialty.

The CORE program has been highly successful. Since 1985, more than $10 million in research funding has been awarded through CORE. Grants range from $5,000 to $70,000 and are 1-year or 2-year, nonrenewable grants. Such seed funding is often critical in developing data that permit a successful application for substantial federal funding.

The CORE study section reviews are similar to NIH reviews. Hence, the process also provides valuable experience and feedback for young investigators who take advantage of this invaluable Academy resource. For example, during 2018, the CORE study sections reviewed 159 applications that requested $2.5 million in funding. A total of $499,902 was awarded to 31 approved grants in various fields of otolaryngology. A listing can be found on the AAO-HNSF website[1] and in the *AAO-HNSF Bulletin*.[2]

Otolaryngologists with good ideas to enhance knowledge and improve our specialty need not be full-time employees in academic centers, and they do not have to be senior, seasoned investigators. The AAO-HNSF is happy to provide not only convenience through the CORE program, but also mentorship. Otolaryngologists should be familiar with this resource and should not hesitate to apply for research funding through the CORE program, and physicians in other specialties that do not have analogous programs should consider initiating them.

References

1. American Academy of Otolaryngology–Head and Neck Surgery. CORE Grants. https://www.entnet.org/content/centralized-otolaryngology-research-efforts-core-grants-program. Accessed August 13, 2018.
2. American Academy of Otolaryngology–Head and Neck Surgery. CORE grants awarded. Partnering to advance the specialty. *AAO-HNS Bulletin* 2018:37(6):20–2.

Reprinted with modifications by permission of Vendome Group from:
Sataloff RT. Centralized Otolaryngology Research Efforts (CORE) grants. *ENT J* 2017;96(8):282.

25. Reg-ent: An invaluable new offering from the American Academy of Otolaryngology-Head and Neck Surgery

We live in a world in which quality of care will be analyzed and used not only for reimbursement, but also for many other purposes. The American Academy of Otolaryngology-Head and Neck Surgery Foundation (AAO-HNSF) developed a new data registry called Reg-ent that should be invaluable for practicing otolaryngologists and might serve as a useful model for other specialties.

The Centers for Medicare and Medicaid Services (CMS) acquires quality data through Qualified Clinical Data Registries (QCDR) that it approves. Reg-ent, an otolaryngology-specific clinical data registry developed by the AAO-HNSF, has been federally approved and is available to AAO-HNSF members. Although there undoubtedly will be implementation challenges as occur with any new computerized system, Reg-ent was very well thought out. In particular, it was designed to be almost effortless for users.

Reg-ent was designed in technologic collaboration with FIGmd (a corporate collaborator) and has a registry practice connector (RPC) that allows it to acquire data from an otolaryngologist's Electronic Medical Record system. It is a read-only link to the otolaryngologist's electronic health record (EHR) that can extract data from the EHR and download it to Reg-ent when the physician's practice initiates a connection session (Reg-ent cannot initiate data collection). The RPC can be installed on a physician's database server, or on a computer that has access to the EHR database.

What good is such a system to the individual physician, and is it safe? From a confidentiality perspective, this system is not only safe but federally approved, and it does not put patient-identified information at risk. However, it does do several valuable things for practitioners.

Physicians are being required to report quality data to the federal government, and the amount of data reporting required is likely to increase. Because Reg-ent has been federally approved as a QCDR, physicians can use it as their CMS Physician Quality Reporting System, and the data reported through this system will be acceptable to the government under the Merit-Based Incentive Payment System.

In addition to providing information to a national data bank, physicians will have access to their own performance data, which will be available with comparisons to national benchmarks. Under current regulations, the AAO-HNSF is allowed to create up to 30 Otolaryngology-Head and Neck Surgery-specific performance measures for quality improvement and reporting. Early users of this system will have an opportunity to influence the evolution of performance measures for our specialty through the AAO-HNSF.

As otolaryngologists, we should be grateful to the AAO-HNSF for its successful efforts in this extremely important initiative. The data acquired through Reg-ent will be helpful in guiding individual physician improvement, and improvement of the specialty overall. Reg-ent also will be able to help track the efficacy and side effects of new drugs and devices. In time, it is anticipated that participating otolaryngologists will be able to use data entered in Reg-ent to assist them in meeting the requirements for maintenance of certification and licensing for the American Board of Otolaryngology and state licensing boards, as well as for other purposes.

More information can be obtained at www.entnet.org[1] and through a listing in the *AAO-HNS Bulletin*.[2]

References

1. American Academy of Otolaryngology–Head and Neck Surgery. Reg-ent ENT Clinical Data Registry – FAQs. https://www.entnet.org/content/regent-ent-clinical-data-registry-faqs. Accessed on September 19, 2018.

2. American Academy of Otolaryngology–Head and Neck Surgery. REGENT^{SM} UPDATE. Quality reporting for 2016. *Bulletin AAO-HNS* 2016,35(5):6.

Reprinted with modifications by permission from Vendome Group from:
    Sataloff RT. Reg-ent: An invaluable new offering from the American Academy of Otolaryngology-Head and Neck Surgery. *ENT J. 2017*;96(4,5):154.

26. Access to quaternary care

Although our health care delivery system is changing, some of the goals behind health care reform over the last decade are likely to persist. One of these is the desire to increase access to care. So far, this has been attempted through control of health care costs, insurance reform, and re-designing the health care delivery system through not only payment reform but also the institution of accountable care organizations (ACOs).[1,2] ACOs were started by the Center for Medicare and Medicaid Innovation and are responsible for the health of specific, assigned populations of patients.[3,4] Payments for ACOs are adjusted based upon results measured months to a year after treatment and directed at assessing the costs and quality of care. The results of these assessments lead to bonuses for providers, or assessments requiring return of funds.[2]

Access to quaternary care is relatively limited. So, for efficiency, and because quaternary care is naturally concentrated in quaternary care institutions such as universities, patients travel longer distances for quaternary care than they do for routine care. The association of long travel times and medical outcomes has been studied in general surgery.

Mehaffey et al.[5] reviewed the outcomes of 17,582 patients treated at the University of Virginia, Charlottesville, Virginia. The median travel time of their patients was 65 minutes, with a median distance of 54 miles. Of this total, 45.5% of their patients were considered local, traveling less than one hour; and 54.5% (9,576) considered regional, traveling more than one hour. The regional group had significantly higher rates of transfer, inpatient surgery, American Society of Anesthesiologists (ASA) classifications greater than two, and rates of several medical comorbidities. They also were more likely than local patients to have non-independent functional status, ventilator dependence, and greater than 10% weight loss in the past six months. Moreover, the regional group had higher predicted risks of 30-day morbidity and mortality in comparison with the local group.

Interestingly, the findings of the study were not entirely what one might have predicted. Despite the higher predicted risks of mortality and morbidity associated with increased pre-operative risk factors, there was no difference in 30-day mortality associated with greater travel time. However, higher rates of prolonged ventilation, re-operation and wound infection were noted, as were significantly higher health care costs. Nevertheless, although 30-day survival statistics in regional patients were comparable to local patients, long term mortality was not. Divergence between the groups occurred by 90 days and persisted over the ten years of follow up of some of the subjects.

Although the study by Mehaffey et al. was single center and retrospective, American College of Surgeons National Surgical Quality Improvement Program (ACS- NSQIP) data were collected prospectively. Even though outcomes for regional and local patients were similar at 30 days, and although the divergence at 90 days and greater might be due to the severity of disease that led patients to travel longer distances, more information is needed to understand the implications of long travel to receive quaternary care, as well as to investigate ways to mitigate differences, possibly through improvements in local follow up care, telemedicine follow up, or other interventions. In addition, similar studies of patients in other specialties should be encouraged, and strategies should be developed to improve access to and outcomes from quaternary care.

References

1. Britt LD, Hoyt DB, Jasak R, et al. Health care reform: impact on American surgery and related implications. *Ann Surg* 2013;258:517–26.
2. Hawken SR, Herrel LA, Ellimoottil C, et al. Understanding pre-enrollment surgical outcomes for hospitals participation in Medicare Accountable Care Organizations. *Am J Surg* 2016;211:998–1004.
3. Ellimoottil C, Miller S, Ayanian JZ, Miller DC. Effect of insurance expansion on utilization of inpatient surgery. *JAMA Surg* 2014;149:829–36.
4. Berkowitz SA, Ishii L, Schulz J, Poffenroth M. Academic medical centers forming accountable care organizations and partnering with community providers: the experience of the Johns Hopkins Medicine Alliance for Patients. *Acad Med* 2016;91:328–32.

5. Mehaffey JH, Hawkins RB, Mullen MG, et al. Access to Quaternary Care Surgery: Implications for Accountable Care Organizations. *JACS* 2016;224(4):525–30.

Reprinted with modifications by permission of Vendome Group from:
    Sataloff RT. Access to Quaternary Care: Studies Needed in Otolaryngology. *ENT J*, in press.

27. Data Scientists: They know what we don't know that we don't know about Big Data

Appreciation of the value of 'Big Data' has increased recently. Our use of Big Data involves secondary analysis of previously published data. This technique permits research involving large numbers of cases using previously accrued primary data; and this approach has received increasing attention.

For example, the American Academy of Otolaryngology–Head and Neck Surgery has facilitated otolaryngologists' access to data sets by creating a resource on the Academy's website, developed through the efforts of the Outcomes Research and Evidence-Based Medicine Committee (OREBM).[1] Initially, the website listed information on a dozen databases of potential interest to otolaryngologists wishing to pursue secondary data analysis, and the list gets updated.

Many of us, including the author (RTS), have published research using some of these databases.[2,3] However, as we increase our use of these important resources, it is prudent to avoid doing so naively and to be aware of expertise that should be at our disposal. It is also important to recognize that Big Data opportunities can involve studying far more than previously published information. A wealth of material is sitting in our records that has not been explored systematically.

As an analogy, most experienced researchers recognize the value of working with an expert statistician. Even those of us with some knowledge of statistics realize the importance of an expert statistician's insights into research design and analysis. In working with Big Data, physicians should be aware that a new profession has evolved that specializes in optimizing Big Data management and can provide insights, consultation, and added benefits in Big Data research analogous to, and in some cases even greater than, those provided by a statistician in traditional research. The new professional is called a data scientist. Given the complexities and potential of Big Data analysis, adding a data scientist to our research team seems at least as important as collaborating with an experienced and creative statistician.

Data science is a relatively new field, as reviewed in a fascinating article by Davenport and Patil.[4] The term data scientist was introduced in 2008 by D.J. Patil, head of analytics and data for LinkedIn, and Jeff Hammerbacher, former head of data and analytics for Facebook and co-founder with Patil of Cloudera, a data analytics company.[4] Data scientists are high-level professionals with expertise in computers and often other scientific fields (such as physics, systems biology, ecology, astrophysics, and others). Davenport and Patil described the data scientist as a 'hybrid of data hacker, analyst, communicator, and trusted advisor'.[4] Essentially all data scientists can write computer code, and most have eclectic understanding of multiple fields. They create tools to bring manageable organization to larger amounts (petabytes) of data, including data that are not organized neatly into rows and columns of numbers.

Big Data science is made possible in part by new technologies such as cloud computing, data visualization, Hadoop for distributed file system processing, and others. The field is exciting, primarily for the brilliance and outside-the-box approach of its practitioners. Data scientists delve into overwhelming quantities of data and create ways to structure huge quantities of unorganized information. They recognize promising data sources, identify and fill in incomplete data, integrate various data sources creating communication abilities among them, and clean and organize the resulting data set.

Even when technology to accomplish their goals is limited, data scientists find ways to cull and organize information from massive data collections. As an example, a data scientist studying fraud recognized an analogy between the fraud problem and a kind of DNA sequencing and was able to amalgamate data management approaches from those two vastly different spheres in order to reduce fraud losses.[4]

Data scientists are being used widely in big business, but they are badly underrepresented in medicine and medical research. Unfortunately, they are also hard to find. When Davenport and Patil wrote their article in 2012, there were no degree programs in Data Science. Now, there are degree programs at major universities in almost every state, but they are relatively new and small. Consequently, being rare assets in short supply, data scientists can be very selective about the environment in which they work.

It is likely to be easier to attract data scientists to an organization with the resources of Google or Amazon than to many medical settings. However, there must be data scientists who are interested in medical research using Big Data; and we should be proactive in inspiring and recruiting them for university programs that train data scientists. Davenport and Patil provided a list of 10 hints on how to find a data scientist, and their article is worth reviewing.[4] Unfortunately, many of us physicians will have trouble understanding the answers to the questions Patil and Davenport suggest posing in the search for data scientists. However, our computer and information technology consultants, statisticians, and other creative scientists and colleagues are likely to be helpful in communicating with and recruiting these invaluable professionals.

The importance of Big Data has become more and more apparent in many surgical fields. For example, in 2015, the Bulletin of the American College of Surgeons (ACS) featured an article 'Big promise and big challenges for big health care data'.[5] In that article, Coffron and Opelka noted the importance and growth of health information technology and its potential for enhancing medical knowledge. They discussed the Health Information Technology for Economic and Clinical Health (HITECH) Act, and the potential importance of and barriers to expanding the use of Big Data in healthcare settings. They called for surgeons to assume active leadership roles to realize the full potential of a data ecosystem.

While the ACS article is correct in most respects, it is open to challenge in its assertion regarding an optimal Big Data ecosystem that 'surgeons have the experience and expertise to create this environment and to use it to improve efficiency and outcomes'.[5] We surgeons need to guard against our tendency to believe that we can do and know pretty much everything. Physicians certainly need to be involved in the process of driving the evolution of Big Data systems and being certain that these systems generate clinically useful data; but we need to be aware of our shortcomings and our need to function as part of a team of experts that includes knowledge and perspective beyond our expertise.

We also need to recognize the need for caution when using or interpreting Big Data. Some of the issues are crystallized nicely in an early article by Tim Harford published March 28, 2014,[6] and brought to my attention by Dr. Brian McKinnon. Harford acknowledged the four primary claims of Big Data: (1) exceedingly accurate results; (2) every data point can be captured; (3) statistical correlation reveals what we need to know, regardless of what causes what; and (4) scientific or statistical models are unnecessary. However, he contended that these claims are 'at best optimistic oversimplifications"

Harford stressed the fact that the many small data problems encountered routinely do not disappear because we have large volumes of data, and they may actually grow worse. He also suggested that the flu trend predictions that heralded much of the enthusiasm for Big Data turned out to be inaccurate. He emphasized that the 'found data sets' used in Big Data analysis contain biases that are difficult or impossible to identify.

Recognizing that the use of Big Data has detractors as well as enthusiasts is essential for physicians. It is yet one more reason that we need expertise beyond our own and that of our traditional statisticians in order to gain as much insight as possible into the strengths, weaknesses, truths, and myths of Big Data. As noted by computer scientist Joshua Lipschultz (personal communication, 2016), 'Conventional statistics and data science alike can yield incorrect results.' Physicians will benefit from association with data scientists in our effort to minimize errors in our own Big Data research and to recognize them in research submitted to our journals for review and in published papers.

Physicians involved in research should be familiar with the young but rapid evolving field of Data Science, and we should make efforts to consult data scientists to help us in optimizing the Big Data sets to which we are turning more and more. The size of our Big Data is tiny compared with the data sets with which data scientists usually work. It is unclear whether that will make is easier or harder to recruit them or for them to enhance our research, but it seems clear that collaboration with experts in this new field should be explored so that the data we want analyzed can be exploited optimally, and so that we avoid misunderstandings about and pitfalls of Big Data research. It is likely that data science professionals will find much more useful information in our Big Data sets than we will on our own.

References

1. Accessing big data for research? A new resource for AAO–HNS members. *AAO–HNS Bulletin*. May 2014:39.
2. Rutt AL, Hawkshaw MJ, Sataloff RT. Laryngeal cancer in patients younger than 30 years: A review of 99 cases. *ENT J* 2010;89(4):189–92.
3. Austin SA, Hawkshaw MJ, Sataloff RT. External ear sarcoma: A review of the Surveillance Epidemiology and End Result (SEER 17) database. *ENT J* 2011;90(8):348–58.

4. Davenport TH, Patil DJ. Data scientist: The sexiest job of the 21st century. Harvard Business Review; October 2012:70–6.
5. Coffron M, Opelka F. Big promise and big challenges for big health care data. *Bull Am College of Surg* (April) 2015:10–6.
6. Harford T. Big data. A big mistake? *Significance* 2014;11(5):14–9.

Reprinted with modifications by permission of Vendome Group from:

Sataloff RT. Data Scientists: They know what we don't know we don't know about Big Data. *ENT J* 2016;95(8):302–5.

Part III: Publication

28. Peer review: Universal, but valid?

The scientific community depends upon peer-reviewed literature. We believe that our prestigious, peer-reviewed journals help ensure that published papers are honest and valid. Most peer-reviewed journals have been stressing the importance of evidence-based research in their various disciplines, and they have understandable biases toward publication of articles that report well-controlled studies with evidence-based results. Surprisingly, there are few such studies investigating the effectiveness of the peer-review process itself.

The peer-review process is not without critics. Many have challenged it on the basis of fairness, accuracy, reliability, transparency and standardization, among other concerns. The peer-review process also has been accused of suppressing creativity, delaying publication, suppressing truly new concepts, and other shortcomings. Nevertheless, it is accepted widely and relied upon by editors, authors, and readers. However, until recently, even the attitude about, and acceptance of, the peer-review process remained unstudied.

In 2008, an interesting survey of the attitudes and behaviors of 3,040 academics in numerous disciplines (medical and nonmedical) performed in 2007 shed light on the current status of peer review.[1] Initially 41,140 surveys were sent; the 3,040 replies constitute an impressive effective response rate of 7.4%. Ninety-eight percent of the respondents were current authors and had published at least one paper during the preceding 24 months. Six hundred thirty-two (21%) were editors, only 14 of whom were not also current authors.

The survey confirmed the overwhelming acceptance of peer review as a valued component of our publishing system. Ninety-three percent of respondents disagreed with the assertion that peer review is unnecessary, and 85% agreed that peer review helps scientific communication greatly. A resounding 90% of the study cohort believed that peer review is effective primarily in improving the quality of published papers, and 89% acknowledged that the peer-review process had improved their last published paper.

Despite these expressions of support, many of the authors and editors surveyed recognized that the peer-review system could be improved. Only 64% of academics were satisfied with the current system; 32% felt that the current system is the best that can be achieved, while 36% disagreed with that assertion. Only 12% identified themselves as dissatisfied with the current system of peer review. A surprisingly small 38% were dissatisfied with the time delays involved in the peer-review process, believing that it is too slow.

Various peer-review techniques are in common use. Many journals use a single-blind review process. That is, the reviewers know who the authors are, but the reviewers remain anonymous. Other approaches are double-blind reviews, open reviews, and post-publication reviews. Only 25% of those surveyed preferred the single-blind review process; 56% preferred double-blind reviews, 13% favored open review, and 5% supported post-publication review. Double-blind review (neither the reviewers nor authors know the others' identities) was regarded as most effective by 71% of respondents. Fifty-two percent felt that single-blind review was effective, with 37% acknowledging post-publication review and 26% recognizing open review as effective.

Despite the support for double-blind review, it has some significant shortcomings. Various problems render it extremely difficult to achieve consistently in practice. For example, experienced reviewers commonly can determine the authors' identity based on subject matter, references, writing style, and other characteristics of a manuscript.

In open review, the identities of authors and reviewers are known. Forty-seven percent of reviewers stated that disclosing their name to the authors would make them less likely to review an article. It is surprising that the number is not higher, and we might suspect that sacrificing anonymity would inhibit the review process severely.

In pure post-publication review, articles are published more or less as they are submitted and critiques are provided with or following publication. Only 5% preferred this approach over the other three approaches discussed above, but 53% agreed that it would be a useful supplement to peer review. At present, the closest that most medical journals come to this process is the publication of Letters to the Editor to point out important flaws that have appeared in print and were overlooked during the peer-review process. Another variant of post-publication review is replacing peer review with post-publication quality ratings or with usage or citation statistics. Fewer than 7% of respondents supported using this approach.

It was surprising that detailed review of the scientific data, statistics, etc., is apparently not a routine and universal component of the peer-review process. Forty-five percent of editors and 40% of reviewers felt that it was not realistic to expect peer reviewers to review an author's data in detail, although 68% of authors and 63% of reviewers felt that it was desirable; and 51% of reviewers said that they would be willing to review the data themselves. These responses also were surprising, particularly in light of the problem of reviewer overload.

Ninety percent of the authors surveyed also functioned as reviewers, reading manuscripts regularly for an average of 3.5 journals and, occasionally, for an additional 4.2 journals. Active reviewers (6 or more reviews in the previous 12 months) completed an average of 14 reviews per year. Hence, active reviewers were responsible for 79% of all reviews. This group expressed a preferred maximum of 13 reviews per year. Considering the entire group of respondents, the average reviewer completed 8 reviews per year and declined about 2 requests to review per year. About 20% of requests for review are declined overall. Not surprisingly, the active reviewers not only complete more reviews but also decline proportionately fewer invitations.

The average review was completed within 4 weeks and took a median of 5 hours. Seventy-six percent of journals used online manuscript submission and tracking.

Editor overload was not really addressed as a problem in that initial survey, but it might be an issue. It was surprising to learn that the average number of papers on which an editor made decisions regarding acceptance or rejection was about 50 per year. The majority of editors (59%) reported handling fewer than 25 papers per year. Only 11% of editors handled 150 papers or more. I found this particularly enlightening, since in 2017 I handled 869 manuscripts as editor (350 for *Ear, Nose & Throat Journal* and 519 for *Journal of Voice*) and more as reviewer, and I found the volume manageable. The average acceptance rate among all journals was 50%, with about 20% rejected prior to review because of inadequate quality or a topic being outside the scope of the journal. Of the 50% accepted, 40% required revisions.

Considering how much work is involved, one might wonder why professionals choose to be reviewers. By far, 'playing your part as a member of the academic community' was the most common reason (91%) in the initial survey study. Others included 'to enhance your and further your career' and 'to increase the chance of being offered a role in the journal's editorial team', but these reasons were much less common. While 35% believed that reviewers should be paid (40% were opposed to payment), the majority acknowledged that paying reviewers would make publication unaffordably expensive.

The complete initial survey by Mark Ware Consulting that has been summarized in this chapter is 73 pages long and can be viewed in its entirety online.[1]

The Publishing Research Consortium repeated surveys in 2009[2] and 2015[3] (published in 2016). Comparing the most recent results with the study performed in 2007 shows interesting consistencies and a few changes. This discussion will compare the 2015 study with the 2007 study. Overall satisfaction (65%) and dissatisfaction (9%) with the peer-review process were unchanged, as was the opinion that peer-review remains necessary to control scientific communication and improve the quality of public papers. Respondents felt that the peer-review process is most effective in improving quality, determining originality and determining the importance of findings. They found it least effective in detecting fraud and plagiarism. Respondents still considered the process desirable and were willing to review data. The number of manuscripts reviewed and declined was similar during the two studies. Respondents felt that there were some improvements over time, particularly improvements in the ability to detect fraud and plagiarism. These might be due to computer programs available to publishers. Interestingly, fewer respondents felt that the system needed to be overhauled completely (26% in 2015, compared to 35% in 2007). The number of respondents who felt that peer-review holds back scientific communication rose from 19% in 2007, to 26% in 2015. In the most recent study, there was no longer a preference for single-blind versus double-blind review; and the percentage of respondents who support open review increased. Interestingly, the number of respondents who cited self-interest as a reason for participating in the review process declined substantially in the most recent survey. There was also a surprising decrease in the number of respondents who declined reviews because of too many reviewing commitments (13% at 2015, compared with 56% in 2007). Most of the other questions listed answers that had no significant change over time.

In 2014, Chetty[4] published a fascinating article studying reviewer behavior. 1,500 reviewers were included, with 2,500 reviews over 20 months in four experimental groups. A deadline of six weeks was used as the control group. When the deadline was shortened from six weeks to four weeks. Reviews were received two weeks sooner with no change in quality. When the four-week deadline was supplemented by a $100 payment if the deadline were met on time, review time was reduced by ten days. When turnaround time was posted publicly, reviews also were received sooner. However, this social incentive was most successful with senior reviewers (tenured professors). This study demonstrated in a most interesting fashion that reviewer performance can be changed by journal policy.

These studies provide interesting insights into the peer-review process as it currently exists and highlight some of the problems and shortcomings that warrant further consideration. They also highlight a disturbing paucity of research and publication regarding the peer-review process itself.

Since current policies determine what gets published, what we read, and how our patients are treated, and since those policies and their efficacy are virtually untested, it seems incumbent upon us to devote more thought to this important aspect of our scientific lives, and to initiate research to determine the best way to evaluate and encourage optimal scientific publication.

Reference

1. Publishing Research Consortium. Peer review in scholarly journals: Perspective of the scholarly community—an international study. January 2008. Bristol, UK: Mark Ware Consulting, Ltd. http://www.publishingresearch.net/documents/PeerReviewFullPRCReportfinal.pdf
2. www.publishingresearch.net/documents/peerreviewfullprcreport-final.pdf
3. Publishing research consortium/index.php/pre-projects/peer-review-survey-2015
4. Chetty R. How small changes can influence reviewer behavior. Journal of Public Economics. Posted on May 1, 2014. https://www.elsevier.com/reviewers-update/story/peer-review/how-small-changes-can-influence-reviewer-behavior. Accessed September 19, 2018.

Reprinted with modifications by permission of Vendome Group from:
Sataloff RT. Peer review: Universal, but valid? *ENT J* 2009;88(4):848–51.

29. The editorial process: Resident and graduate student education and participation

In September 2005, the *Ear, Nose & Throat Journal* editorial board agreed to create a new opportunity for resident education. Two positions on the editorial board were created for residents, each of whom was to serve a two-year term. This plan was introduced in an editorial I wrote in the journal in January 2006. We have been pleased with the experience, and this chapter presents a review of our initial concept, reflects upon the early results, considers ways to improve the process, serves to remind residents that editing opportunities are available, and seeks to encourage other journals to consider adding residents to their editorial boards.

The motivation for this experiment is reiterated here. The advancement of medical science and clinical care depend on publication of valid, relevant papers. Traditional medical school education and residency training incorporate little or no formal instruction in techniques of writing publication, journal selection, publication ethics, or the editorial process. In addition to teaching medical trainees how to write, we have found it extremely valuable to provide them with editorial training. Such training improves an individual's writing, as well as his/her ability to judge published works.

The lack of formal training in basic writing skills is a matter of concern. Training in a variety of specific writing techniques should be included as a required component of residency training, but that is a subject for another discussion. Editorial training is even less common, but it is exceedingly valuable to physicians, even those who might have no interest in serving on an editorial board, because it provides important information that improves an individual's writing and ability to judge the value of published works. Editorial board training includes learning about incisive, analytical reading and critique of literature, but there is a great deal more involved. Editors and reviewers also need to understand medical ethics, the definitions of duplicate publication (which are not always obvious and which change over time), political and economic issues that can affect publication (and might not always be apparent at the time of the initial reading of a submission), the nature of conflicts of interest and their potential impact upon published results and clinical practice, the complexities involved in standardizing nomenclature, and many other topics of interest and importance to the scientific and clinical evolution of medicine.

Participation on an editorial board gives a resident an opportunity to develop analytical skills not only by reviewing manuscripts, but also by reading reviews prepared by expert, experienced members of the editorial board. Serving as Editor-in-Chief of *Journal of Voice* and *Ear, Nose & Throat Journal* has provided me with an intriguing education. After more than three decades as an editor, I am still fascinated by the process. I read manuscripts, make judgments, send them out to world-class reviewers, and learn an enormous amount by reading their insights and seeing the manuscript again from a different perspective. Members of the editorial board enjoy a portion of this educational benefit when we 'cross review' (send reviewers each others' comments on a given manuscript). We do so routinely when there are substantial disagreements among the reviewers. Our resident editorial board members review manuscripts that also are reviewed by the usual number of editorial board members, and the resident editors generally are supplied with the comments of all of the other reviewers. This process was designed to let the residents learn what they might have missed.

Our experience over the first two years was favorable, and to make it even better, in 2008 we increased the number of resident editorial board positions from two to at least four. The initial reviews by the excellent residents selected for membership on the editorial board were of high quality and occasionally provided valid insights that augmented the reviews of our regular editorial board members. The process was enhanced further by including formal discussion and training at the annual editorial board meeting about the form and components of a good review. This discussion includes not only the resident editors, but also the established members of our editorial board. We believe that this discourse is not only educational for the resident members, but also that it improves the quality and consistency of reviews from the entire editorial board. We launched a similar initiative with the *Journal of Voice* in 2010. However, because of its multidisciplinary nature, we included graduate students as well as residents. The results were excellent with both journals; and many of the residents/student reviewers have become full members of the editorial board following completion of their training programs.

In 2014, we believed that the resident-editors program at *Ear, Nose and Throat Journal* had been in place long enough to justify asking the nine residents who had served on the editorial board about their experience.[1] All nine responded to a questionnaire. Three of the residents had attended an annual editorial board meeting, and all found it interesting and useful. All nine reported having found their experience on the editorial board interesting and educational and said that the experience made it more likely they would serve on an editorial board in the future. Five of the nine residents planned careers in academic medicine, two were unsure, and two planned other career paths. All nine said that they wanted to continue as members of the *Ear, Nose, and Throat Journal* editorial board after completing residency.

Eight of the nine resident editors reported that the number of manuscripts that they had been asked to review was 'just right', and one felt he/she had not been asked to review enough manuscripts (most resident reviewers are asked to review about 10 manuscripts per year). They all felt that the turnaround time required for reviews was 'just right' (2 weeks).

Three residents suggested that the experience could be enhanced by more contact with other reviewers, perhaps by assigning a mentor from the editorial board to each resident editor. They felt that more feedback would be helpful. One reviewer suggested that the residents might be invited to help rewrite (for a small fee) manuscripts written by authors whose native language was not English.

All of the residents who have had the opportunity to serve on the editorial board have found the experience beneficial and rewarding. Interestingly, reviewer ratings of the resident editors ranged from 82.5 to 90. Reviewer ratings were assigned to resident reviewers in exactly the same manner in which they were assigned to the other editorial board members. The resident reviewer performance exceeded that of some of our regular editorial board members.

In the summer of 2016, under the guidance of Jack Krouse and Cecelia Schmalbach, the journal *Otolaryngology–Head and Neck Surgery* launched an excellent related initiative called the Resident Reviewer Development Working Group (RRDP). This project brought interested PGY-3 residents together with outstanding, experienced reviewer mentors. The 1-on-1 association allowed for deep, critical and detailed analysis of residents' reviews, and tailored plans for improving knowledge and editing ability. The RRDP will undoubtedly enhance resident knowledge and future availability of well-educated reviewers.

Including residents on our editorial boards has provided unique and valuable opportunities for the residents and graduate students to participate in the editorial process and it has highlighted opportunities to improve editorial board education in general. We believe that including residents and students helps them in their preparation to become leaders in academic medicine and other fields, and we suspect that the information that they carry back to their fellow residents and students expands the impact of this educational experiment beyond those who are actually selected for editorial board membership. I believe that this experiment has been successful and will become even more successful as more journals established similar programs. I encourage editors of other journals to consider adding resident and graduate student members to their editorial boards.

References

1. Sataloff RT. Resident editors. *ENT J* 2009;8(7):984–6.

Reprinted with modifications by permission of Vendome Group from:
Sataloff RT. The editorial process: Resident education and participation. *ENT J* 2008;87(7):364–5.

30. Correcting the medical literature: Ethics and policy

Editors and publishers take their responsibilities seriously. There are international congresses on peer review in biomedical publications, many of the most important contributions from which are published in classic, special issues of *Journal of the American Medical Association (JAMA)*. A wide range of topics is discussed, including the nature of peer review, whether reviews should be anonymous, whether reviewers should be blinded to the identity of the authors, techniques to minimize publication bias, ways of dealing with plagiarism, the impact of fraudulent research on scientific literature, the effects of institutional prestige and author nationality on reviewers' recommendations, and many other topics.

While the importance of correcting medical literature after fraudulent publication has been addressed, surprisingly little attention has been paid to the important issue of correcting the medical literature after publication of bad papers. The peer-review process is intended to detect poorly designed or misleading articles before they are published. The process is flawed, however; and substandard articles can appear in any journal.

Editors try to avoid this unfortunate occurrence in several ways. Usually, we assign submitted manuscripts to more than one reviewer, and we select reviewers who should be knowledgeable about the subject matter being reviewed. Moreover, we encourage our reviewers to decline manuscripts that are outside their areas of expertise and to suggest alternate or supplemental reviewers. For example, it is common for reviewers to request that a manuscript receive additional review by a statistician, to be certain that no subtle errors go unrecognized, especially if such errors might affect the validity of the conclusions.

Despite our best efforts, once in a while we publish something that should not have been published. Hence, it is surprising that so little attention has been paid to the obligation of a journal to acknowledge this situation and correct the literature when correction is warranted.

In an unusual practice that might be unique to our field, otolaryngology journal editors meet twice a year at the Combined Otolaryngology Spring Meeting (COSM) and at the American Academy of Otolaryngology–Head and Neck Surgery (AAO-HNS) meeting. There, we discuss a variety of subjects ranging from standardization of terminology to the problem of duplicate publication, but this issue has not been on our agenda. I suspect that most of us have assumed that such corrections are handled adequately through letters to the editor, editorials, or retractions. However, addressing such issues occurs at the discretion of the editor in most cases. So, response to such events varies.

This problem was highlighted for me more than a decade ago through my correspondence with the *Journal of the American College of Surgeons (JACS)*, certainly a deservedly well-respected publication. In October 2004, *JACS* published an article on voice changes after thyroidectomy.[1] While being delighted to see an article on voice in the College's journal, I was dismayed at its quality. The clinical examinations were not sufficiently sophisticated to meet the current standards of clinical care, let alone those of clinical research. No blinded, subjective analysis of the clinical data was included. Preoperative and postoperative laryngeal electromyographic data were not provided, so the status of laryngeal nerve function remains unknown. The voice-analysis system used is not particularly sophisticated, and details of recording protocols were not provided. Also, the parameters selected for reporting were inappropriate. The analysis program used generates data on a variety of other measures, but this paper excluded those data and provided no information as to why they were excluded.

Perhaps more importantly, the errors in the data reported in that article are profound in their naiveté. For example, shimmer was described as a measure of intensity. This is completely inaccurate. Shimmer is a perturbation measure that describes cycle-to-cycle amplitude variation and has no predictable correlation with vocal intensity. Intensity should be measured in decibels SPL under carefully controlled conditions.

This article was fatally flawed and would not have been accepted in any otolaryngology journal. Immediately after the article was published, I wrote a letter to Timothy J. Eberlein, M.D., Editor of *JACS*, and I received an admirably prompt, standard rejection letter indicating that the rejection 'usually reflects issues of timeliness, a backlog, or beliefs that the material, when complete, did not fit our readership'. I would have accepted this outcome happily if my letter had been rejected because another letter had been accepted and was to be published to point out the shortcomings of the article, by Sinagra et al. However, follow-up contacts with the journal indicated that this was not the case. Hence, readers of *JACS*, most of whom are not sophisticated in their analysis of voice literature, are likely to believe the unsupportable conclusions stated in that article. For otolaryngologists who read other voice literature, this may not be a problem; but for thyroid surgeons who read primarily general surgical literature and who may rely on that article, it is a problem.

Readers of all journals should be aware not only that the peer-review process is imperfect, but also that the ethics and policies involved in a journal's response to the publication of bad literature have not been discussed widely or standardized, and that the response of any journal when such issues arise may lie in the hands of one person. Editors are well-meaning, but we are not always expert in the subject matter of every paper published in our journals. Also, we are faced with numerous pressures regarding journal space and other matters, and we are not blessed with (or bound by) standard policies or guidelines that help determine our response when the validity of a published article is challenged.

These facts highlight not only the need for all of us to read critically, but also the need for more formal review of this subject by publishers, editors, and ethicists interested in optimizing the peer-review process and the quality of medical literature.

References

1. Sinagra DL, Montesinos MR, Tacchi VA, et al. Voice changes after thyroidectomy without recurrent laryngeal nerve injury. *J Am Coll Surg* 2004;199:556–60.

Reprinted with modifications by permission of Vendome Group from:

Sataloff RT. Correcting the medical literature: ethics and policy. *ENT J* 2005;84(2):65–6.

31. Publication as a teaching tool

While the importance of publication is recognized widely within the academic community, even those of us who publish extensively are surprised occasionally by the value of publication to our teaching mission. I thought that I had learned most of what there was to know about the teaching value of publication. However, the thirty-ninth book I wrote proved me wrong.

Various aspects of publication have obvious, well-established teaching merit. Medical students and residents writing their first papers learn to organize information (and their thoughts, in the process), recognize and eliminate extraneous information, review literature in an organized fashion, and express themselves articulately. In doing so, they develop greater expertise in the subject of their paper. They also commonly have opportunities to present the topic orally, helping them learn how to teach others in accessible language.

As faculty edit and correct students' papers, the trainees improve their skills. Moreover, as their publications become more complex, they learn to analyze and synthesize more voluminous and complex information, honing their intellectual acumen. Incisive critique from faculty, statisticians, and other mentors increases their expertise. By the time trainees finish residency or graduate school, publication training also has increased their ability to think concisely, express themselves well, and recognize shortcomings in publications that they read.

Editorial experience also has great teaching value. Inviting residents to review manuscripts submitted to journals, for example, challenges them to evaluate experimental design, presentation, validity and reliability. Sharing with residents the critiques of experienced reviewers who have assessed the same manuscript provides invaluable training. However, although I have recognized and appreciated the teaching value of publication for decades, and although I have always used trainees' drafts of papers as an opportunity to evaluate and teach them, I did not appreciate fully the potential of publication as a method for assessing training until spring 2010.

Like many in the medical profession, I have trained residents and fellows for many years. At the conclusion of residency training, our impressions from direct observation, along with standardized test performance, generally give most of us the feeling that we have a reasonably valid perception of our trainees' knowledge. This is also true with fellows, even though standardized examinations are not available in all fellowship subjects. Nevertheless, I work extremely closely with my laryngology fellows on a daily basis, and by the time they have graduated, I have been confident that they knew what I expected them to know. My most recent publication experience has not only shown me that I was wrong, but it also has provided me with an opportunity to fill knowledge gaps.

Along with two co-authors, my laryngology fellow and I completed the *Atlas of Endoscopic Laryngeal Surgery*.[1] This book includes numerous intraoperative photographs of voice surgical procedures. Toward the end of the fellowship year, I asked my fellow to write the first draft of the figure captions and the first draft of the detailed steps describing the sequence of each surgical procedure. He was an excellent fellow, one in whom I have substantial confidence.

As expected, most of what this fellow wrote was correct. However, much to my surprise, there were key misunderstandings and several subtleties (rationales) that were omitted. Since he was an excellent technician and since I thought I had covered most of these subtleties during the course of the year, I had not anticipated finding any substantive errors in his writing (although I expected to refine the language). To the contrary, this publication exercise ended up serving as an extensive 'final examination' of the details and fine points of endoscopic laryngeal surgery. It revealed what he did not know (that is, what I had not taught him adequately) and gave us an opportunity to review in detail every maneuver and concept of laryngeal surgical technique.

The experience was invaluable for both of us. It allowed him to recognize and correct areas of misunderstanding, and it taught me that even the best of my graduates might not know everything that I think they know. That experience has made me even more thorough in my teaching, and it has led me to look for new techniques to assess knowledge of surgical procedures. In retrospect, I wish I had asked all of my former fellows to write a similar atlas, and certainly look for opportunities to assign equally revealing tasks to current and future fellows.

Publication is invaluable to advancing the field, but it is also an unmatched educational activity. Even those of us who publish extensively and require our trainees to publish extensively should reconsider the potential contributions of publication to our educational programs and should continue looking for new ways to make publication even more valuable, not only to our readers but also to our authors.

References

1. Sataloff RT, Chowdhury F, Joglekar SS, Hawkshaw M.J. *Atlas of Endoscopic Laryngeal Surgery*. New Delhi, India: Jaypee Brothers Medical Publishers, 2010.

Reprinted with modifications by permission of Vendome Group from:
Sataloff RT. Publication as a teaching tool. *ENT J* 2010;89(10):478–9.

32. Journal ethics: Let the reader beware

Most authors, editors, journals and publishers are committed to honesty, transparency, and ethical conduct. As readers of medical literature, we depend on that commitment, and we have a tendency to assume that it exists. Unfortunately, that is not always the case.

At the level of an author or researcher, all of us are aware of the problem. Safeguards have been enacted to help identify and prevent commercial bias. Conflict of interest information is solicited, and authors sign forms identifying potential conflicts or attesting that none exist. Blatant dishonesty and failure to declare conflicts of interest are uncommon, but not unheard of. Occasionally, undeclared conflicts are uncovered during the peer-review process by editorial board members who may be aware of conflicts that were not acknowledged. Although a problem may slip through occasionally, reasonably good systems are in place to protect readership against undeclared conflicts and commercial bias.

While most of us are alert to such problems, we are less likely to think of them with respect to entire medical journals. It is disturbing to know that problems can occur at the journal level, even with journals published by an extremely experienced and respected publisher. Perhaps the most infamous example involves six articles appearing between 2000 and 2005 in journals published by Elsevier. This scientific publishing giant is justifiably highly respected and publishes approximately 2,000 medical journals worldwide - including *Journal of Voice*, which I edit (consider that a disclosure).

In that instance, the *Australasian Journal of Bone and Joint Medicine* published what was essentially a collection of reprinted scientific articles and in one article, published reviews that were highly favorable to products of the pharmaceutical company Merck & Co., Inc. The articles were published under Elsevier's *Excerpta Medica* imprint, and they gave no indication that the publication had been paid for by Merck.

Similar problems occurred in other publications from the Australian office of Elsevier's *Excerpta Medica* imprint, including the *Australasian Journal of General Practice*; the *Australasian Journal of Neurology*; the *Australasian Journal of Cardiology*; the *Australasian Journal of Clinical Pharmacy*; and the *Australasian Journal of Cardiovascular Medicine*, in addition to the *Australasian Journal of Bone and Joint Medicine*.

When the problem was discovered, Elsevier responded appropriately and made efforts to ensure that proper use of disclosure language would appear in any future publications, and such problems have not been identified in Elsevier's hundreds of other medical journals. However, the information about undisclosed sponsorship may never reach many of the readers of these publications who might reasonably assume that they had read unbiased, peer-reviewed articles and might rely on them for the care of their patients.

While such publishing misconduct is probably rare these days, even in the 21st century it has not been eliminated completely. Physicians should be familiar with this additional potential source of bias, especially when reading journals with which they are not familiar. Critical reading is necessary not only to evaluate scientific design and validity, but also to be certain that conclusions are not tainted by commercial or political bias.

Reprinted with modifications by permission of Vendome Group from:
Sataloff RT. Journal ethics: Let the reader beware. *ENT J* 2011;90(1):8.

33. Case reports in medicine

Clinical observation has been the basis of advances in medicine since at least the time of Hippocrates. Although case reports have fallen into disfavor among academicians and editors in recent years, a review of literature from the 20th, 19th, 18th, and 17th centuries (and before) reveals case reports to be the intellectual foundation upon which modern medicine was built. Case reports tell the stories of our patients and stimulate our imaginations. Much of what we know and use to treat our patients was learned through case reports. This tradition has enriched all specialties of medicine and is responsible for our early understanding of everything from vaccination to stapes mobilization to heart disease. Physicians still like to learn through the clinical experience of colleagues and do so through informal discussion, grand rounds, and other venues. However, wide dissemination of clinical insights through publication of case reports has become more and more difficult.

There are two primary reasons why it is hard to get case reports published. The first is the current enthusiasm for evidence-based medicine (EBM).[1] The impetus behind that enthusiasm is admirable. As a profession, physicians should be concerned about assuring that published information is valid and reliable. Clinicians often use published reports as guides to patient treatment. Hence, we must admire efforts to be certain that published papers are of high quality. The rigors of EBM help promote validity and reliability, although they certainly do not assure the accuracy of all published papers. Inaccurate manuscripts still slip through the editorial process; but the growing awareness of the importance of EBM helps emphasize the need for critical analysis and scrutiny of every article we read. It also provides a structure to help evaluate an article's credibility. However, evidence-based, placebo-controlled, double-blind trials are not the only writings worthy of publication in the medical literature. Much can still be learned from sharing clinical experience through single case reports or, better, through case series that illustrate practical aspects of clinical encounters, novel observations, new treatment approaches, and perplexing questions. Such publications should be viewed by readers differently from excellent evidence-based studies. Readers need to exercise extra judgment in determining the credibility of such articles and how they should be applied. Case reports do not (and should not) pretend to put forth scientifically proven universal truth. Rather, they attempt to share information and provoke thought, questions and further communication and study.

The second reason why it is difficult to get case reports published is (embarrassingly) pragmatic. Through their publishers and editors (I am currently Editor-in-Chief of two traditional peer-reviewed medical journals), journals strive for credibility. Credibility improves the prestige of a journal, attracting high-quality authors, as well as advertisers. One of the measures of a journal's prestige is its 'impact factor'. Impact factor is determined by calculating how often articles published in a journal are cited by indexed journals. For example, to determine a journal's impact factor, the number of articles published by journal X in 2016 and 2017 that were cited by indexed journals in 2018 is divided by the total number of citable publications (articles, reviews, proceedings) published in journal X during 2016 and 2017. Case reports lower a journal's impact factor. If a journal publishes a first-reported case of a condition (regardless of how interesting that report may be), it may be 20 years before someone finds a second reported case and cites that article. Sadly, many editors and publishers have yielded to these pressures and have decreased drastically the number of case reports that they are willing to publish.

Case reports and case series offer useful and thought-provoking information that at a minimum allows clinical teaching (in a sense, bedside mentoring) to achieve worldwide reach through publication, and at best inspires thought and dialogue among readers that will lead to additional case reports and series, more formal research, and greater knowledge.

Case reports are a critical compliment to EBM, and together they form the substance from which the next generation of medical advances will evolve.

References

1. 1.Sataloff RT. Evidence-based medicine. *ENT J* 2006;85(10):624–5.

Reprinted with modifications by permission of Vendome Group from:
Sataloff RT. Case reports in medicine. *ENT J* 2013;92(8):324–6.

Part IV: Politics

34. Healthcare for the uninsured: A simpler, cheaper, faster, better solution

There are a great many problems in the United States associated with access to healthcare, not the least of which is the fact that the terms *healthcare* and *health insurance* have become nearly synonymous to the public. Fundamental conceptual flaws in our paradigm for healthcare payment are worthy of consideration. However, altruism and recent legislative debates require that we first consider our most pressing problem: the best way to care immediately for Americans without health insurance. Most physicians agree that a country as wealthy as the United States should have some system to protect our citizens who have essential health needs that they cannot afford. However, solving that problem has led to extremely contentious debates, legislative proposals that threaten to bankrupt the country, and coverage 'requirements' that many consider inconsistent with the principles of democracy and capitalism (and which might even be unconstitutional). The proposals, debates, and posturing suggest that they are driven by political agendas rather than by a pure commitment to caring promptly for our uninsured population, since there seems to be an obvious solution that apparently has not been entertained seriously.

First, let us consider the real magnitude of the problem. When ObamaCare was put forward, the best available numbers were based on the most recent U.S. census.

According to that census report, in 2007 there were 45.7 million people in the United States without health insurance.[1] However, this number bears closer scrutiny. Wenger summarized important subsets of those census data:

- 14 million of those uninsured were below the poverty threshold and were eligible for Medicaid, but they had failed to apply for Medicaid.
- 11 million had declined health insurance offered to them by their employers because they elected not to spend the portion of their pay required to cover the employee contribution.
- 18 million of the uninsured had a household income of more than $50,000 per year; and, interestingly, 9 million of those had a household income of greater than $75,000 per year.
- 9.7 million of the uninsured were illegal immigrants.[2]

It was pointed out that 70% of the uninsured people in the United States actually have access to health insurance but have elected not to obtain coverage.[3] Let us take a conservative look at the real number of uninsured who reasonably may be considered for care at taxpayers' expense through a new approach, based on numbers that were obtained based on our historical norms prior to the enactment of ObamaCare. Certainly, we can subtract the 14 million Medicaid-eligible Americans from the 45.7 million. The system is already prepared to cover them, and all they have to do is apply.

I would also contend that we should subtract the 11 million people who have declined health insurance from their employers. The United States is a democracy. If people elect to gamble by not insuring their homes, their cars, or their health when they have the ability to do so, that is their right. If they choose to run the risks of being uninsured in order to be able to spend their money on something else, they are exercising freedom of choice but must also accept responsibility for the consequences of that choice. If that decision leads to the loss of a home or a lien against future earnings in a democratic society, then so be it. There is no reason why taxpayers should be obligated to bail out what essentially amounts to a lost gamble.

Even eliminating only those groups, the number of uninsured drops to about 20.7 million. Arguments can be made about whether the 9.7 million illegal immigrants or 9 million with household incomes exceeding $75,000 a year should also be subtracted (there is some overlap in some of the groups defined above). However, even without addressing these groups, the magnitude of the problem is clearly not quite as overwhelming as the numbers usually bandied about by politicians.

If the President were to decide tomorrow that his real and only immediate concern were to provide basic and emergency healthcare access to the legitimate uninsured who need it right now, is there a way to do that cost-effectively and expeditiously? I would argue that we already have an excellent federal healthcare system in place that could be used to ameliorate the crisis without disrupting the healthcare system, forcing through incompletely considered and contentious legislation, or instituting or perpetuating nondemocratic (socialist) 'reforms'. The Veterans Administration (VA) is an excellent, generally well-run, widely distributed federal healthcare system that, with augmentation, could care for the uninsured population and would cost far less than any of the proposals that have been considered.

The VA has the nation's largest integrated healthcare system, with 172 comprehensive medical centers and approximately 1,062 outpatient clinics distributed throughout the United States, where care is provided to more than 9 million veterans annually.[4] The VA healthcare system is organized into 21 regions called Veterans Integrated Service Networks (VISN). Each is responsible for coordination and oversight of all administrative and clinical activities within its region.

In 2009, the VA had approximately 270,000 full-time equivalent employees and more than $100 billion in obligations.[4] In providing healthcare to veterans and their dependents, with 5.6 million unique patients in 2009, 99% of primary care appointments were completed within 30 days of the requested appointment date, and scores on Quality of Health Care performance evaluations are high and improving.[4] The VA also has the nation's largest and most sophisticated telehealth program, which already provides care for 230,000 patients in more than 144 VA medical centers and 450 community-based outpatient centers.[4] By 2019, the funding request increased to $198.6 billion. Among other tasks, these funds will support 366,358 full-time equivalent employees. It is anticipated that 7 million patients will be treated in the VA Hospital System during 2019. Mental health services are anticipated to provide 15.2 million outpatient visits, and the total number of outpatient visits in the VA System in 2019 is anticipated to be 118 million. Pension benefits will be provided for approximately 269,000 veterans and 200,000 survivors.

To put utilization into perspective, the estimated population of veterans in the United States (not including dependents who also may be entitled to VA Hospital benefits) is about 23,400,000.[4] With the VA's proven track record of efficiency and excellence, it seems as if it would make much more sense to expand VA services and provide a prompt, efficient solution to the problem, rather than trying to reinvent healthcare financing in the United States. In addition, even if the VA Hospital budget were doubled or tripled, the expenditure would be far less than the trillion-dollar budgets discussed in Washington.

I believe that if the federal government gave the VA Hospital systems the financial resources required and called upon the VA to rise to the current need, that the essential health needs of the legitimate uninsured could be handled easily, almost immediately, and without any adverse effect on the care provided to veterans. In fact, the influx of resources to enhance the VA system would probably benefit veterans.

Moreover, if additional physician resources were needed and our federal government were capable of thinking outside the box, recruiting volunteer physicians would not be difficult, either. If the government provided physicians with malpractice coverage for their activities in the VA system (equivalent to the malpractice coverage provided to employed VA physicians), and if the government offered physicians a tax credit for their activities at VA hospitals equal to the amount that they customarily *bill* for those activities in their normal settings, it is likely that a great many physicians would volunteer their time for a day or two a month, if needed. Their presence also would enhance treatment available to our veterans, in addition to providing coverage for the uninsured. Customary billing amounts are easily verifiable through the previous year's submissions to health insurance carriers. Admittedly, health insurance carriers don't use the billing numbers for much other than calculating the 'adjustment' column, but they do have the numbers that could be used for verification to avoid abuse of the system.

This proposal could be implemented quickly, and the uninsured who need healthcare would have a place to go long before our legislators finish debating and implementing the sweeping health financing reforms repeatedly under consideration. To be sure, our system of financing healthcare deserves reform, but taking care of our uninsured should mean more than using them as leverage to revamp our entire healthcare system or influence elections. If the powers-that-be really care about the health of uninsured Americans, they should open the doors of our federal VA healthcare system to them now, and not hold them hostage to philosophical debate and political wrangling.

References

1. Income, poverty, and health insurance coverage in the United States: 2007. Washington, D.C.: U.S. Census Bureau; August 2008. Available at: https://www.census.gov/prod/2008pubs/p60-235.pdf. Accessed November 2018
2. Wenger RD. Does the U.S. have the best health care system in the world? *Bull Am Coll Surg* 2009;94(7):8–15.
3. Gratzer D. *The Cure: How Capitalism Can Save American Health Care*. New York: Encounter Books; 2006: 81–100.

4. United States Department of Veterans Affairs. http://www.va.gov/. Accessed August 22, 2018.

Reprinted with modifications by permission of Vendome Group from:

Sataloff RT. Healthcare for the uninsured: A simpler, cheaper, faster, better solution. *ENT J* 2010;89(2):52–5.

35. Undermining market forces: A fundamental flaw in American healthcare

As physicians, many of us are living in a world we could not have imagined 30 years ago. We entered medicine expecting to dedicate our lives to helping people, we anticipated that our dedication would be appreciated and our efforts would be reasonably well rewarded socially and economically. Instead, our ability to practice medicine is hampered by 'gatekeepers' whose responsibility is to maximize the profits of insurance companies, not the welfare of patients. Their frequently uninformed decisions determine what care an individual may receive, and although they affect treatment directly, they are protected from legal action that would hold them responsible for these decisions.

In addition, Americans in general have developed an extraordinary sense of entitlement regarding healthcare. Not only do American consumers demand the best healthcare, but many seem to believe that it should be free. There is no interest in cost-effectiveness with regard to one's own personal healthcare and patients are often prepared to litigate if any information is missed or delayed in its discovery. How did we get in this mess? Each of the issues above is worthy of a chapter, but this chapter will focus only on the last issue.

One of the principal reasons that healthcare costs have become (arguably) problematic is that market forces have been largely removed from the practice of medicine. The insurance model in medicine is unique. In any other setting, if an insured event occurs, a person pays for a service and is then reimbursed by his/her insurance company (or signs over insurance company reimbursement to the provider). For example, if one is in an automobile accident, the driver finds a body shop that he/she selects based on expertise, cost, convenience, and other factors. The insurance company inspects the car and determines what it considers reasonable reimbursement. The driver interacts directly with the body shop and is responsible to the body shop. The driver also deals directly with his/her insurance company, as owner of the policy.

In medicine, it no longer works that way. The patient, who is the owner of the policy, is essentially not in the loop (except perhaps for a co-pay or 'deductible' expense). This allows insurance companies to deal directly with doctors - a small group with notoriously ineffective lobbying. This might seem like a small issue, but it is not. Patients are voters. To illustrate, if the patient were paying for a service, he/she would select a doctor based on expertise, cost, convenience, and other factors. The patient would then see the doctor and be presented with a bill. Let us say that the bill was $100. The patient would recognize that as reasonable, feasible, and fair for the services rendered and pay it. If the patient received $85 from the insurance company that would probably be acceptable. If the patient received $20, after having paid insurance premiums, he/she would probably find that unacceptable. The patient would then contact the insurance company, perhaps the insurance commissioner, perhaps the press, and perhaps his/her congressman. Market pressure would be applied to keep insurance company reimbursements reasonable, and the voting public would keep the system in reasonable balance. It would be easy enough to create contingencies for patients who are not able to provide reimbursement in advance of insurance payments, but for most people such an arrangement (using cash or credit) would be easily manageable for most medical encounters.

Such an arrangement (which is the usual arrangement for insured services in anything except for medicine) would have the added advantage of making patients aware of healthcare costs. Americans are exceptionally demanding of the healthcare system. I believe this is good; it has resulted in remarkable advances in medicine and a high standard of care. However, Americans demand the widest possible choice of physicians and hospitals,[1] the shortest waiting time in the world for elective surgery,[2] unlimited access to cancer screening and treatment, even though it might not extend life significantly (especially from a societal standpoint),[3] essentially unlimited access to advanced diagnostic imaging and other tests, unlimited access to healthcare for the elderly and those who are terminal, and other uncompromisingly comprehensive healthcare treatments, regardless of cost.

This attitude may not be unreasonable, but it is hard to judge it when the patients do not bear the costs and are not involved even temporarily in paying for the costs. In many cases, they do not even know what the costs were. Furthermore, those Americans who discuss cost-effectiveness generally do not understand that much of the time they are talking about accepting missed or delayed diagnoses in order to save societal expense. They vote for cost-effectiveness but sue for delayed diagnosis. For example, if we order an MRI every time there is a 20-dB high-frequency asymmetry in hearing, occasionally we will diagnose an acoustic neuroma when it is extremely small, but we will have ordered a great many negative MRI studies. If we wait a year or two until the hearing gets worse (or some other symptom develops) and then order a MRI, that may be more cost-effective, but the doctor will be at risk of litigation for failure to diagnose the tumor a year or two earlier.

When patients think about these issues in the abstract, eliminating 'unnecessary' studies sounds good. When they are sitting in the office talking about their personal MRI, their analysis usually is different. Under many insurance plans, the MRI will cost them nothing other than, perhaps, a modest co-pay. Since there is little (if any) expense to patients, when it comes to their personal health they are not interested in cost-effectiveness, they are interested in knowing whether they have a tumor now, not a year or two from now when it has grown larger.

The solution to this part of our health problem couldn't be simpler. Restore capitalism and market forces to medical care. The voting public has managed to maintain most other segments of the economy pretty well without excessive regulatory interference from Washington. The government's current laws and plans for medicine promise to make this fundamental flaw in the healthcare paradigm even worse than it already is. Our nation has rarely gone wrong putting faith in voters rather than government. I believe that restoring market force controls would work well for healthcare delivery, too.

References

1. World Health Organization. The World Health Report 2000. Health systems: Improving performance. Geneva, Switzerland: World Health Organization, 2000. http://www.who.int/whr/2000/en/whr00_en.pdf. Accessed September 20, 2018.

2. Ohsfeldt R, Schneider JE. The business of health: The role of competition, markets, and regulation. Washington, DC: AEI Press; 2006.
3. Lai DJ. Measuring the impact of HIV/AIDS, heart disease and malignant neoplasms on life expectancy in the USA from 1987 to 2000. Public Health 2001;120(6):486–92.

Reprinted with modifications by permission of Vendome Group from:

Sataloff RT. Undermining market forces: A fundamental flaw in American healthcare. *ENT J* 2010;89(9):408–10.

36. Healthcare system failure: A planned strategy?

In 2010, I read an article[1] that discussed an issue I planned to address in a chapter. It is probably written better than what follows, and it is certainly much longer and more detailed than our page limitations permit. In it, Dr. David Cossman analyzed the U.S. government's intrusion into healthcare, focusing on the implications of the Patient Protection and Affordable Care Act (PPACA). He speculated insightfully about the U.S. government's intention to take over healthcare. I reached similar conclusions, some of which I will highlight in this chapter, but I believe that Dr. Cossman's article still is worthwhile reading for all of us, even though the federal healthcare landscape might be changing. It also might change back!

These issues have great potential impact on healthcare in general, but also on subspecialty care and clinical research. All physicians have benefited from the advances achieved through the traditional paradigm of medical practice in the United States. The opportunities for creative practice and independent financing of clinical research and treatment evaluation have led to remarkable advances in many specialties. We must consider how a major change in the business of medicine will affect our ability to provide world-class care, and to advance medical knowledge and care.

PPACA is long, complex, and probably unmanageable. It appears to me that even the federal government must have recognized its shortcomings and could not blame them all on compromise. It made me wonder whether the administration really believed that all of the problems could be addressed in the execution, or whether the new healthcare system was actually expected to fail. I was uncertain whether ObamaCare's intrinsic flaws were due to legislative incompetence/political expediency, or something more Machiavellian.

Dr. Cossman made a strong case suggesting that the bill was 'designed intentionally for failure because the architects were sore that they had to remove the public option and wanted to throw healthcare into chaos to expedite a second run at a federal takeover'. I had reached the same conclusion, and Dr. Cossman's cogent argument solidified that belief.

There are many flaws in ObamaCare legislation, but some of the most glaring highlight the reasons that it was almost surely destined for failure. The law added about 32 million patients to insurance rolls. The insurance companies surely benefited, but could the medical system provide the care that Americans have come to expect?

The law contains virtually none of the critical support to permit implementation. There are no additional funds for establishing new medical schools, training more physicians, or even increasing the funding for postgraduate medical training. There is no provision for more interns and residents to help create enough physicians to care for the increased volume of patients. Not only are there no funds to increase reimbursement for physicians forced to care for a greatly increased number of patients, but the government actually cut physician reimbursement to help make the new healthcare law appear as if it were revenue-neutral.

There also was a Medicare tax increase of 3.8% on investment income, but there is nothing that allows physicians to either decrease their overhead costs while maintaining quality or raise fees to compensate for increasing overhead. The bill also did not eliminate the sustainable growth rate calculation for physician payments. It easily could have helped physicians by subsidizing physician extenders, forgiving medical student loans (particularly since the government has now gone into the student loan business), or other measures.

At the same time, the bill created approximately 150 new agencies, boards, and other organizations, and called for 250,000 new federal employees to staff them at an estimated cost of approximately $1 trillion. Like most federal financial projections, we can expect this to be an underestimate over time, if repeal of the law or substantial changes do not occur. Moreover, this is far more bureaucracy than is needed to enable private insurers to cover more patients or to monitor the process.

However, if a bureaucracy that size should already be in place and already budgeted when the government decides to impose a single-payer system, it might be very handy for our 'friends' in Washington. They might even use this massive federal structure to argue that a single-payer system could be implemented at no additional cost in federal bureaucracy.

So, what can we expect? Dr. Cossman and I have reached the same conclusion. I believe that we can expect the current effort to fail, and I think we can expect the government (over time and mitigated or aggravated by whomever is in power at any given time) to use the resulting chaos and disappointment to try to take over healthcare. Many physicians are likely to try to address this problem by dropping out of the insurance system, becoming either nonparticipating physicians or concierge physicians. However, if we think that this safeguard will work, we are being profoundly naïve politically.

The government's most likely response would be to force us by law to treat every patient who walks through the door. Impossible in a free society, you say? If you think so, ask your local hospital CEO. The Emergency Medical Treatment and Active Labor Act (EMTALA) already requires hospitals to care for anyone who shows up in the emergency room. Requiring physicians to do the same thing will not seem like such a big step on Capitol Hill. There are already states with laws that have moved in that direction, although not globally. For example, in Pennsylvania, it is illegal to charge, or accept from, a Medicare-eligible patient any more money than Medicare would have paid, regardless of whether the physician participates in Medicare (Medicare Overcharge Measure, 35 P.S., Section 449.33). However, it is still possible, although onerous, for physicians to refuse to treat patients who are eligible for Medicare. So far, I am not aware of any physicians who have stopped seeing Medicare patients, but if enough chose that strategy, the response might well be a law precluding us from doing so.

We and our patients are in trouble, and there is reason to believe that it is going to get worse. As Dr. Cossman pointed out, 'Takings are supposed to be illegal'. However, there is reason to worry that the government is headed toward seizing our intellectual property and ability to control our profession. If PPACA is any example, we are unlikely to even be compensated (as we would if the government seized our land by eminent domain). We are likely to be expected to continue paying for our own education, overhead, malpractice costs, and all of the other expenses of medical practice, and yet have the federal government limit not only our incomes but also our abilities to choose how we practice and whom we treat. Perhaps the Supreme Court might determine that this federal approach is unconstitutional (challenges already have been raised); but there is little sympathy for, or understanding of, our position and concerns among the voting public. So, when the federal government tries again to dismantle traditional American medicine, remove it from the free market, put it under federal control, and assure the voting public that this is the solution to affordable care, there is a chance that the government will succeed. Sadly, by the time patients realize what this means in terms of quality care and physician attention, it will be too late.

We need to recognize the dangers now and do everything that we can to protect freedom of medical practice before more damage is done. That includes being much more generous with political action committee contributions than we have been traditionally, and it includes supporting politicians who understand the importance of free market forces and physician independence in the U.S. healthcare industry. Our traditional system has created extraordinary advances in medical care. These have resulted in the development of world-class subspecialty care in many fields, and major discoveries through research funded not only federally but also privately through healthcare revenues and corporate support. Virtually all subspecialties of medicine have evolved through scientific and technologic advances made possible through the traditional approach to medical practice. These advances have helped not only patients in the United States, but also doctors and their patients throughout the world.

There are many ways to provide healthcare for everyone in the United States without dismantling the uniquely successful tradition of medical practice. We have been too quiet for too long. If we do not step up and intervene now, it may be too late sooner than we think.

References

1. Cossman DV. The Taking. *General Surgery News* 2010;37(10):1,40–2.

Reprinted with modifications by permission of Vendome Group from:

Sataloff RT. Healthcare system failure: A planned strategy? *ENT J* 2011;90(9): 404–6.

37. Price controls in medical practice

Most physicians choose to participate with health insurance carriers, but most physicians have no real choice. In order for most doctors to opt out of participation with third party carriers and still maintain financially viable practices, essentially all of the other local physicians in their specialty would have to do the same. As we all know, there are legal impediments against physicians even gathering to discuss such collaborative actions, let alone the specifics of reasonable fees. The only exceptions are truly unique or extraordinary doctors who provide services not available elsewhere, or who limit their care to patients who can afford concierge medicine.

At present, what constitutes a 'reasonable' fee is defined by insurance companies and applies to virtually all physicians in an area (perhaps with a small adjustment for physicians employed full-time in an academic institution). If you own a basketball team and hire Lebron James, you do not pay him the same salary as you pay the average college graduate who just joined the NBA. Yet, if I perform microlaryngeal surgery, I receive the same reimbursement as a general otolaryngologist who finished residency last year. Neither Medicare nor private insurers distinguish highly experienced from newly minted practitioners.

Both for this reason and because of the continual threats regarding cuts in Medicare reimbursements, there has been increased discussion about doctors changing their status regarding Medicare, if not other carriers. However, the decision not to participate in Medicare is more complicated than it may seem, especially in light of a peculiar law in Pennsylvania that bans 'balance billing' Medicare patients, even by physicians who choose not to participate in Medicare. While physicians in most other states are not burdened with similar laws, several states have already enacted comparable bans and more certainly might. It is worth reviewing physicians' three options regarding Medicare.

First, a physician can participate (PAR) and accept Medicare assignment. In that case, the physician is paid 100% of the Medicare fee schedule (80% by Medicare and 20% by the patient or a supplemental insurance carrier). Second, the physician can be nonparticipating (non-PAR). In this case, the patient is paid 95% of the Medicare fee schedule (80% of which comes from Medicare and 20% of which comes from the patient or supplemental insurance). The decision to participate or not can be made on a case-by-case basis. In most states, if physicians are non-PAR they can bill patients up to 115% of the Medicare fee schedule. However, that is illegal in Pennsylvania and several other states (see below).

The third option is opting out of Medicare altogether. This approach cannot be made on a case-by-case basis. In order to opt out of the system, the physician needs to leave Medicare for at least a two-year period. This requires signing an affidavit agreeing to receive no payments from Medicare during that time. Each patient also must sign a contract prior to receiving any services from the physician stating clearly that the patient gives up all Medicare payment for those services, will not bill Medicare or ask the physician to bill Medicare, and will be liable for all of the physician's charges without any Medicare balance-billing. The patient also must acknowledge both that Medigap and other supplemental insurance will not pay for the services, and that he/she has been advised that services can be received through other physicians from whom Medicare coverage is available. The contract cannot be entered into when the patient is facing an emergent or urgent health problem.

While these requirements are quite burdensome, it remains unclear whether complying with them, at least in Pennsylvania, will actually enable a physician to enter into a private contract with a patient at mutually agreeable, negotiated fees.

In 1990, the Commonwealth of Pennsylvania enacted a law (35 PS Section 449.33). This legislation outlaws balance billing a Medicare beneficiary. That is, whether a physician is PAR or non-PAR, it is illegal to charge any Medicare beneficiary 'an amount in excess of the reasonable charge for the service provided, as determined by the United States Secretary of Health and Human Services'. A challenge to the ban by the Pennsylvania Medical Society was rejected by the United States Court of Appeals for the Third Circuit in 1991 (Pennsylvania Medical Society v. Marconis, 942 F2.d842 [3d Cir. 1991]), so the ban still applies. Thus, while in most other states, non-PAR physicians are able to balance bill, they are not permitted to do so in Pennsylvania. Since this onerous law has been upheld, physicians in all states are at risk of facing similar legislation.

It remains unclear how this Pennsylvania statute affects physicians who opt out of Medicare entirely via private contract, in accordance with the federal opt-out law. On the one hand, as worded, the Pennsylvania law might be interpreted as applying even to physicians who opt out under the federal law, since the law specifies that it applies to any Medicare beneficiary. On the other hand, the federal opt-out law was enacted in 1997. Because it was enacted after the Pennsylvania law and its purpose was to ensure access to medical care for Medicare beneficiaries by giving patients and physicians the freedom to contract outside of Medicare, it might be argued that the federal opt-out law supersedes the Pennsylvania law, so that the Pennsylvania ban against balance billing Medicare patients doesn't apply to physicians who opt out in accordance with the federal law. Thus, the situation in Pennsylvania and other states with similar laws remains uncertain; at present, it is unclear whether physicians who opt out of Medicare in accordance with the federal law will be able to charge and collect fees any greater than Medicare would have paid if they had been participating.

As the federal government becomes more aggressive about removing market forces and freedom from healthcare, more and more physicians are likely to reconsider their decisions to participate with various insurance carriers, including Medicare. In most jurisdictions, doctors still have the freedom to make that choice, thus enabling them to negotiate their fees with their patients. Especially in the current political climate, we should remain vigilant. We must be aware of all legislative initiatives that further impinge upon our freedoms and those of our patients, as well as our obligation to preserve the business of medicine in a manner that will sustain our ability to provide our patients with optimal medical care.

Acknowledgment

The author is deeply indebted to Martha Swartz (mswartz@swartzhealthlaw.com), a healthcare attorney whose contributions and insights were invaluable in the preparation of this chapter.

Reprinted with modifications by permission of Vendome Group from:
    Sataloff RT. Price controls in medical practice. *ENT J* 2010;89(11):516–8.

38. Tort reform: Federal impetus for change

Physicians have been active in helping to assure that patients have access to expert care. It is essential that we remain familiar with changes in the healthcare delivery system so we can have input as new regulations evolve, and so that we can adapt to changing programs. It is also important that we recognize not only the shortcomings of legislative proposals, but also the strengths.

Many of us had reservations about the Patient Protection and Affordable Care Act (PPACA), passed into law in March 2010 (and subject to continuing challenges). However, many people agree that it contained some good provisions. Most physicians support the notion that our nation's population should have access to healthcare (although we differ in opinion as to how that aim should be achieved); most of us agree that eliminating the preexisting condition restriction is good; and most of us are in favor of allowing children to remain covered under their parents' policy beyond graduation from college. However, many people are not aware that the law also addresses, at least to a modest degree, malpractice costs. It established a $50 million demonstration program that allows states to experiment with alternatives to the prevailing process for managing medical liability; $50 million is a small amount in a legislation that cost more than $1 trillion, but at least it is something.

Under the PPACA, the Department of Health and Human Services is empowered to award grants to states, enabling them to establish and assess new approaches to dispute resolution and tort litigation. These experimental programs must attempt to improve access to prompt and fair resolution of disputes, improve access to liability insurance, improve patient safety, and encourage disclosure of medical errors. Creating this program suggests that the lawmakers who were in control of the legislature when the law was enacted recognized the need to do something about the malpractice problem, even though they have consistently opposed caps on noneconomic damages as a solution. Although the success of caps in Texas and California does not seem to convince these legislators that caps are a good approach, it is encouraging to know that at least some effort to address the problem was funded in the law.

It is also interesting to note that the Obama administration provided additional grants within its medical liability reform and patient safety initiative. In June 2010, the administration awarded nearly $20 million for seven demonstration grants, six of which focused on patient safety. Although that initiative is admirable, it does not address the needed tort reform directly. New York State received $3 million for the only grant that tested a new approach to handling malpractice claims (a negotiation program directed by a judge). Encouragingly, the administration also provided an additional $3.5 million for planning grants to support the development of projects to reform medical liability processes.

Data from the American Medical Association (AMA) confirm that the malpractice crisis is still with us. According to an article written by Carol K. Kane and published on the AMA website, as of 2011, approximately 65% of malpractice claims filed against physicians were dismissed or withdrawn without payment, and 90% of malpractice cases that went to trial resulted in verdicts in favor of the physician (no negligence).[1] The article also said, 'Average defense costs per claim were $40,649, ranging from a low of $22,163 among claims that were dropped, dismissed or withdrawn, to a high of over $100,000 for tried cases'.[1] These numbers are put into greater perspective in light of additional AMA data showing that as of 2010 an average of 95 medical malpractice claims were filed for every 100 physicians in the United States.[2] More recent data were available through 2016.[3,4] At the time of this writing, patterns across specialty, age and gender were similar to those reported by Kane in 2010 (2007-2008 data).[1] Thirty-four percent of all physicians have been sued, with 16.8% having been sued two or more times and 2.3% being sued in the last 12 months.[3] Psychiatrists and pediatricians are the specialists least likely to be sued and men are more likely to be sued than women.

Several states have initiated efforts to address this perplexing problem. They will not be reviewed in detail in this chapter. However, one approach requires further thought and debate within the scientific community in general; and it may even warrant prospective action. In the state of Oregon, a project was initiated that focused on the use of clinical practice guidelines to establish the legal standard of care. The PPACA advocated use of evidence-based research. The Oregon-proposed law would theoretically support that initiative by legislating that a physician who used best practice guidelines would be able to use the practice guideline as a defense if he/she were sued for an alleged problem arising from that care.

This concept sounds good. The problem is that the vast majority of what we do is not evidence-based. Hence, even when we make a good-faith effort to develop valid guidelines, we depend on opinion in many cases because high-quality evidence does not exist. Ideally, the opinions are expert and well vetted, but even with the best of intentions that is not always the case. Nevertheless, it is likely that we will be called upon more and more to develop clinical guidelines and practice parameters not only to improve medical care and to satisfy third-party carriers, but probably also to help minimize our liability. If that prediction is correct, it is important for us to waste no time in developing the best guidelines and practice parameters that we can, recognizing and codifying that there are legitimate reasons for physicians to deviate from such guidelines for select individual patients.

The process of guideline development brings into sharp focus our deficiencies in evidence-based data. The process should be used to provide appropriate disclaimers in the practice guidelines, acknowledging components that are based on opinion rather than high-level evidence. It also should be used to identify and prioritize research that is needed to develop evidence on which revised guidelines can be based. Funding sources should be encouraged to support such projects, and our legislators should be approached about creating new sources of federal funding specifically to support evidence-based research initiated to address scientific deficiencies identified in the process of developing practice guidelines.

I do not believe that addressing these issues will provide adequate tort reform. The $250,000 caps on noneconomic damages passed in Texas and California have demonstrated that such caps are effective; and we should continue to support legislative initiatives to establish caps. However, it also would be wise for us to become familiar with other approaches to reforming the liability process, and especially to establish quickly a substantial number of well-considered guidelines for care of nearly all disorders, as well as prospective research projects to improve our body of evidence-based research.

References

1. Kane CK. Medical liability claim frequency: A 2007–2008 snapshot of physicians. American Medical Association. http://www.ama-assn.org/resources/doc/ health-policy/prp-201001-claim-freq.pdf. Last accessed June 9, 2011.

2. Medical Center. Malpractice threat to physicians pervasive, AMA study finds. August 6, 2010. http://www.mednewscenter.com/malpractice-threat-to-physi- cians-pervasive-ama-study-finds.htm. Last accessed June 9, 2011.
3. Guardado JR. Medical Liability Claim Frequency Among U.S. Physicians. American Medical Association's Policy Research Perspectives 2017; https://www.ama-assn.org/sites/default/files/media-browser/public/government/advocacy/policy-research-perspective-medical-liability-claim-frequency.pdf. **Accessed September 22, 2018.**
4. Kane, CK. Updated data on physician practice arrangements: physician ownership drops below 50 percent. American Medical Association's Policy Research Perspectives 2017–2; https://www.ama-assn.org/sites/default/files/mediabrowser/public/health-policy/PRP-2016-physician-benchmark-survey.pdf. Accessed September 22, 2018.

Modified from Sataloff RT. Tort reform: Federal impetus for change [Editorial]. *ENT-J* 2011; 90(7):290–2. Republished by permission from Vendome Group.

39. The Board of Directors

Many physicians have been 'leaders' since childhood. The excellent performances that helped many of us earn medical school acceptances include positions as student council members, yearbook editors, sports team captains, and other activities in which our tendencies to excel led us into positions of influence. Hence, it is not surprising that many physicians achieve positions of leadership not only in medical settings but also in community, philanthropic, and political venues.

Despite our busy professional schedules, physicians are appropriately honored when asked to assume leadership roles, and especially to join the board of directors of a prestigious organization. Although these positions are time consuming and often pro bono, we accept such invitations routinely because we enjoy contributing as leaders and because we feel some obligation to share our wisdom and insights. Physicians should be encouraged to accept invitations to boards of directors to which they can make substantive contributions, but we also should be aware of the commitments and liabilities associated with such positions.

Having served on the boards of numerous organizations including medical societies, hospitals, nonprofit philanthropic foundations, and other organizations, and including positions as board chairman, I have come to believe that the time, effort, and risks are well worth accepting; but I also have come to believe that most of us do not understand fully what we are getting into, at least when we join our first board. This chapter is written to review some of the relevant considerations, and it draws not only on my own experience but also on a well-organized exposé on this topic written by Dr. Michael McArthur.[1]

Before accepting an invitation to join a board of directors, it is important for the physician to understand the nature and purpose of the board, what he/she might be able to contribute, and what the expectations of membership are. It is also important to find out who his/her fellow board members will be and to read the mission statement of the organization in order to be certain that the physician is comfortable with (ideally enthusiastic about) what the organization does. It is useful to understand the structure of the organization, as well.

Most boards of directors or trustees are involved in oversight of an organization's management, activities, and governance. Ordinarily, a board does not manage directly. Nevertheless, it is responsible ultimately for the organization under its purview. Potentially, individual board members can be held liable for adverse or illegal activities. Therefore, it is also important for the physician to be certain that the organization maintains directors' and officers' insurance (D&O) that will protect board members in the event of a legal action.

Legally, members of a board of directors have a duty of impartiality, a duty to make the entity productive, a duty of care and a duty of loyalty.

The duties of impartiality and loyalty are related somewhat. A rather oversimplified explanation of these duties is that they require that all decisions and actions be based solely on the best interest of the organization and that no consequences to individuals and entities outside the organization should bias the board member's input to the board. This is not always as easy as it sounds.

Members of most boards are required to declare potential conflicts of interest and to recuse themselves when a conflict or the potential perception of a conflict arises, but it is not always easy for physicians to be impartial. For example, sometimes, as members of a hospital board, physicians participate in debates establishing policies that are good for the hospital but might be financially undesirable for selected members of the medical staff, potentially including the board members and their associates.

A conflict can also arise if physician leaders serve on boards of more than one organization and they come to possess confidential, proprietary information from a board meeting of one organization that might impact another organization in which they hold a leadership role. However, while acting as a board member for an organization, the physician's sole concern and dedication must be to that organization, and it is legally and ethically incumbent upon the physician to recuse himself/herself or resign from a board if such impartial loyalty becomes impossible.

The duty to the make the entity productive is exercised through the board's oversight of all aspects of the organization's activities, and its governance of the organization. The nature and definition of 'productivity' varies somewhat from organization to organization. It may include educational productivity, research accomplishments, global expansion, and other outcome measures; but it almost always includes financial solvency. This is every bit as true for nonprofit organizations as for for-profit organizations, as anyone knows who has sat on a nonprofit hospital board or a 'non-profit' insurance company board.

Maintaining financial viability of the organization is a key board responsibility. Moreover, failure to do so, and the resulting dissolution or bankruptcy of an organization, often has severe consequences - not only for the organization's employees, but also for the community. Such failures routinely trigger government scrutiny and legal inquiry. It is essential for each member of the board of directors to exercise and document due diligence with regard to the organization's affairs, to have the competence to exercise such diligence, and to require that the organization share with the board the information needed in order for the board to govern.

The duty of care requires that the board member monitor the affairs of the organization, and that he/she exercise good judgment and care in all decisions and actions affecting the organization. This duty requires the board member to (1) attend meetings of the board and committees to which he/she is assigned; (2) understand all topics presented to the board; (3) understand the organization itself; (4) have access to and read the financial statements (particularly the annual audit, but also ongoing profit and loss statements, cash flow and budget statements, statements of loans to the organization, and statements about the financial condition of the organization that are distributed to persons outside the board room such as the general public); (5) participate in being certain that the organization is acting legally and ethically; and (6) participate in ensuring that the organization complies with all internal revenue obligations.

Nearly all boards on which physicians are likely to serve are subject to external scrutiny. The primary responsibility of each member of the board is to make certain that the board and organization behave in a matter such that the organization can withstand such scrutiny. Board members will be held accountable (sometimes individually) for the organization's failures (and sometimes for successes). Board members are obligated to be certain that an organization complies with all local, state, and federal regulations and laws.

While it is common for attorneys to be members of boards, or at least available as consultants to boards, it is wise for physicians to develop some familiarity with pertinent laws and regulations if they intend to serve as board members. For example, board members of nonprofit organizations should be aware of some of the more common, seemingly benign, activities that may be violations and may jeopardize an organization's nonprofit status. These include certain kinds of fundraising activities that the Internal Revenue Service defines as for profit.

Another activity that can be problematic for nonprofit organizations is allowing the organization to accept charitable contributions on behalf of a staff member (who may be responsible for having secured the contributions but does not have nonprofit status), if those contributions are not being used directly by the organization. This is called 'acting as a conduit' and while it seems reasonable and appropriate to the mission of an organization, such proposals require legal consultation by the board to determine whether they are legal in each individual case.

Each board member also must help ensure that the actions of the board are transparent. This means that all board actions, activities and decisions must be documented clearly and accurately so that any appropriate party can understand exactly what the board has done, why, who receives compensation (in any form), and how much. The board itself and each individual board member are deemed accountable for the proper exercise of all of these obligations and duties.

To facilitate and document accountability, most boards not only seek out and document conflicts of interest, but also establish various policies to define expectations and activities. These include expectations and documentation of time commitments, development of a policy for ethics and conduct, personnel policies, and financial audit policies and responsibilities.

Serving on boards of directors, trustees, or governors is gratifying and certainly justifies the time and risk. It is important for physicians to share their perspective and insights with medical organizations, and with community, artistic, political, and other entities. However, physicians should recognize the nature and importance of the responsibilities of board membership and of having a commitment to the organization and its cause. It is also important to ascertain in advance that the board members function in a cooperative, collaborative environment, or to recognize any dominant conflicts and controversies and understand them before the physician accepts board membership.

Physicians should be encouraged to accept board membership and enhance their leadership influence, but they also need to understand that serving as a board member is complex and requires thought, education, and commitment.

Just saying, 'Yes, I will do it,' is not sufficient.

References

1. McArthur MS. Physicians and surgeons as board trustees: Be careful what you wish for. *Bull Am Coll Surg* 2010;95(10):26–8.

Reprinted with modifications by permission of Vendome Group from:
Sataloff RT. The board of directors. *ENT J* 2012;91(10):410–2,416.

40. Politics: Getting involved

All physicians in the United States are affected directly and profoundly by politics. The same is true for physicians in many other countries. Hopefully, the thoughts in this chapter will be applicable elsewhere, but they are directed primarily toward those of us who live and practice in the United States.

Over the past several decades, most physicians have observed changes in our practice environment that we regard as changes for the worse. Malpractice litigation in many states has reached troublesome, even crisis, status. In some areas, such as southeastern Pennsylvania, the costs and unpleasant atmosphere associated with an excessively litigious environment have combined with extremely poor reimbursement to create a significant disincentive for young physicians who might otherwise choose to live in such areas. In Philadelphia, for example, despite the attraction of an extremely livable and affordable city - as well as the richness of an academic community with five medical schools - recruiting has become difficult. Furthermore, some excellent, established physicians have chosen to leave the region. Here and in many other cities, the practice environment is made more challenging by other factors, as well, including the intrusions of managed care companies into medical practice, increasing government involvement in patient care through 'pay for performance', electronic medical records, and other initiatives and factors that were far from the minds of most students when they chose to devote their lives to careers in medicine. These problems affect not only the quality of our lives and practices, but also hinder our ability to deliver first-rate care to our patients.

So, how did we end up in this mess?

In the first sentence of the previous paragraph, I noted that we have 'observed changes' and I would argue that that is part of the problem. Most of us went into medicine because we wanted to take care of patients. If we had wanted to go into politics, we probably would have gone to law school. Nevertheless, the past few of decades should have taught us that we cannot afford the luxury of passivity. If we do not become involved actively in the political process, we will continue to be on the receiving end of decisions and policies that affect us and our patients, but over which we have had little or no influence. Since these decisions clearly affect patient care, we have an ethical responsibility to become involved, at least for the protection and safety of our patients if not for other reasons.

We already have spent too much time on the sidelines, trusting that our altruism and dedication would be appreciated and would lead the public to protect us and our ability to practice, but this strategy has failed. For example, numerous surveys have shown that the public has a negative attitude toward physicians, even though respondents have a positive attitude toward their own physicians.

So, once again, how did we get into this mess? There are far more reasons and complexities than can be summarized in the space of a brief chapter. However, I suggest that there is one simplistic and obvious problem that I have never seen discussed elsewhere, and so I will raise it here: television. At the moment, physicians clearly do not enjoy public sympathy and do not hold public confidence to the extent that we deserve. Hence, we are not a potent political force. Legislators have little to gain by supporting pro-physician causes at the expense of alienating other constituencies. When did we lose our public base? It appears to me that it was when Marcus Welby, M.D., Ben Casey, and Dr. Kildare went off the air. They were the last television shows that really developed physicians' characters in depth and showed their dedication and humanity.

Whether we like it or not, a huge percentage of Americans are raised in front of television sets. They get their ideas, images, and stereotypes from the tube. They have enjoyed decades of sympathetic shows about lawyers, ranging from *L.A. Law* to *Law & Order*, but what have they had to watch that helps them appreciate, admire, and strive to emulate physicians? I suspect that if the AMA had spent our money developing pilots and lobbying for network television shows that showed physicians the way we really are, we would have the power of the public and not be in the politically challenged situation that we face now. While this is only one of the causes of our current situation, I believe that it has been largely unrecognized, and its importance should not be underestimated.

Nevertheless, we need to accept our current reality and work proactively to improve it. That means getting involved. Perhaps a few of us have the talent to write some good screenplays and create a hit series about an admirable physician, but for those of us with less writing talent, at the very least we should become involved with the political process, both monetarily and personally.

Many of us complain about the influence of trial lawyers, but it is also well known among politicians that they are lucky to get a $50 contribution from a physician, while a litigation firm is happy to write $10,000 checks to support campaigns. Campaigns cost money, and we can hardly blame politicians for paying attention to the people who help them get elected. Therefore, we need to step up to the plate and support the politicians who support us, our patients, and our beliefs.

As past president of the Pennsylvania Academy of Otolaryngology–Head & Neck Surgery and as an elected Republican committeeman, I would encourage generous support, but I have been surprised at how much even a little bit of financial support is recognized and appreciated. Physicians' political action committees (PACs) provide state and national politicians with smaller contributions than many other PACs (because, unfortunately, we doctors have not been very generous in our contributions to the PACs). However, even at the current, meager contribution levels, politicians notice and appreciate the support, and they listen to our input. More generous support would be better, but contributions from 100% of us (even if some were minimal) would make a striking impression.

Fund-raising events held at our homes for candidates whom we admire also make an impression; one needs only to call the campaign office and offer to hold one, and the candidate's staff will provide assistance. Brief, thoughtful letters to state and federal representatives are welcome and often are read, but personal meetings are clearly better. They can be arranged by appointment with our legislators' local offices; or (sometimes better) they can be facilitated by inviting legislators to speak at events for potential voters and contributors or arranged through faculty associations, county or state medical societies, or independently.

Active participation in the political process is valuable. Although I traditionally have had little interest in politics, several years ago I decided that if I were going to continue complaining, I had better actually do something. So, I ran for committeeman. Committeeman is as grassroots as you can get, and it is a pain in the neck having to go door-to-door every four years to get signatures on the reelection petitions. However, I have learned a great deal about the political process and about my neighbors, and I have been astonished about how much attention senior politicians (even U.S. senators) pay to elected officials even at the committeeman level—and even when the senator is in a different political party. Taking the trouble to participate not only educates us but also gives us credibility in the political process that far exceeds what we would expect for so minor a role.

The suggestions above are easily within reach of all of us in medicine. So is one more: the ballot box. The percentage of people who vote remains embarrassingly low in our great democracy. So low, in fact, that the winners are often determined by whose supporters actually take the trouble to come out and vote. Every election has an impact on us and our patients. There is simply no excuse for any one of us to be observers in the electoral process. If we don't at least show up at the polls, we have little right to complain about what 'they' do to us next.

It has never been more clear that the future of medicine and the care of our patients depend on what happens in state capitols and in Washington. It is high time for us to have our say before decisions are made, rather than complaining about policies after they are foisted upon us. No matter how busy we are, and no matter what our political beliefs, we can no longer afford not to take the time to be involved in the political process.

Reprinted with modifications by permission of Vendome Group from:
 Sataloff RT. Politics: Getting involved. *ENT J* 2006;85(11):690.

41. Politics: Be part of it

For years I complained about all of the lawyers in politics. Over a decade ago, I started sounding disingenuous even to myself. I decided to either be quiet (a daunting challenge) or step up to the plate. So, in 2001, I ran for committeeman. That is the lowest, most grassroots, and least time-consuming elective office I could think of. I have continued to hold it through several election cycles (not that there has ever been any competition); I have found it surprisingly educational.

I believe it is important for physicians to pay attention to legislation and political activity. The actions of state and federal legislatures control our ability to provide high-quality medical care. If we don't express opinions and monitor proposed legislation, then laws will be enacted without our input, and we will have to live with them. If we have opportunities to influence laws for the better and do not take the trouble to exercise those opportunities, then we do not evoke much sympathy or carry much weight when we complain about the results. Hence, I assumed that being part of the political process, even at such a low level, would provide insights.

A committeeman helps support candidates (in some cases helps select candidates), helps get out the vote and works at the polls on Election Day. When I first sought this position, I assumed that I would get to know a few candidates casually, particularly candidates for local and state offices. It never occurred to me that being a committeeman was a 'big deal' in anyone's eyes. After all, the constituents in my precinct number only about 1,000 voters. However, I was wrong. I have had friends for decades who were career politicians, including people in the state legislature and the U.S. Congress.

I was astonished to find that these politicians looked at me completely differently (and listened to me more attentively) when they found out I had become a committeeman. I still am not sure whether that is because professional politicians understand the importance of every dollar and every vote, or because people who hold any elective office (however modest) are part of the process; but there is no question that my election enhanced my access and credibility. In addition, I have gotten to know more politicians at various levels better than I had anticipated.

Talking with local, state, and national candidates (including those who belong to both parties) has been very educational. They have shared ideas, concepts, and political rationale personally while chatting at home or at the polls, as well as at relatively intimate meetings of committee people. I have learned to understand them better and to appreciate (if not always agree with) how they think. I have been able to share with them ideas, concepts, and problems important to all physicians; and I believe some of them even altered their opinions and broadened their vision based on some of these discussions, and their legislative actions have been more insightful than they might have been otherwise.

I have also learned through my service as a committeeman, and through my service as president of and council member for the Pennsylvania Academy of Otolaryngology–Head and Neck Surgery (PAO–HNS), not only the importance of financial support for political candidates and causes of importance to physicians and our patients, but also the fact that the financial support does not have to be extremely high. Before I got involved with elective office and with lobbying through the PAO–HNS and other organizations, I thought that contributions in the thousands of dollars were required to have any impact, or to be noticed and heard by state politicians. It is certainly true that generous contributions are helpful (as the trial lawyers know well, for example), but a contribution of even a few hundred dollars from an individual or society's political action committee is appreciated, noticed, and remembered by politicians.

This does not mean that we can buy physician-friendly and patient-friendly votes. It does mean that the politicians who regulate our lives listen more to people who are involved actively in the political process as office holders, or at least contributors, than they do to people on the sidelines.

Holding even the most basic of elective offices has been unexpectedly gratifying, educational, and politically effective. The commitment requires surprisingly little time except on election days. I would encourage other physicians to get off the sidelines and into the fray.

Reprinted with modifications by permission of Vendome Group from:
  Sataloff RT. Politics: Be part of it. *ENT J* 2013;92(3):98–100.

42. Establishing federal laws

It has become particularly clear in recent years that federal law can have profound influence on the daily practice of medicine. Consequently, physicians have become more active in supporting legislators and legislation that advance efficient, high-quality medical care and patient safety. As we recognize the importance of advocacy in order to have an effective impact on future legislation, it is useful for physicians to understand the processes involved in establishing laws in the United States Congress.

Each year, approximately 6,000 bills are introduced in Congress, although only about 500 (8%) are passed and become law.[1] In Congress, a bill gets started by being written by a member of Congress, usually with the assistance of congressional staff. At any time during the congressional session, the written bill is placed in a box on the rostrum in the Senate or the Speaker's desk in the House. The box is known colloquially as the hopper. A bill number is assigned, beginning with 'S' for a Senate bill and 'HR' for a bill in the House of Representatives.

Once a number has been assigned, the bill is referred to the appropriate committee or committees. There are 19 standing committees in the House and 16 in the Senate. At that point, the influence and expertise of the sponsor (the bill's primary author) are of particular importance. A sponsor who cares about the bill generally makes efforts to enlist cosponsors from both parties, and to communicate with members of the relevant committees. Such efforts are critical, since most bills are tabled in committee. Hence, they are never addressed and 'die' in committee.

Considerable political effort is required even to have the bill debated in committee rather than ignored. In the House, the Speaker may set a time limit after which a committee is required to report back on a given bill, but this prerogative is not exercised for most bills. The entire House also can rescue a bill from committee and have it debated on the House floor through the filing of a 'discharge petition'. To be successful, a discharge petition requires a majority vote of 218 members of the House.

If a sponsor is successful in getting a bill heard before the relevant committee, the bill often will be referred to subcommittees for more intensive analysis. The subcommittee may make changes in the bill. When the subcommittee is satisfied with the wording, a vote is held. If the bill is passed in subcommittee, it is referred back to the full committee. If it does not pass in subcommittee or committee, it is likely to go no further and die. If it is passed in committee, the House or Senate has the opportunity to debate the bill and vote on it.

The process for debate and voting differs in the House and in the Senate. In the House, the House Rules Committee determines when a bill will be considered by the full House of Representatives, how long the debate will last, and how many amendments may be considered. Importantly, in the House, debate and amendments must be relevant to the topic at hand. Hence, some action usually occurs.

The process is different in the Senate. The decision on if/when a law will be considered rests with the Senate Majority Leader. Perhaps most importantly, Senate debate does not have to be relevant (germane). Hence, open-ended debates may result in filibuster, which can prevent a bill from ever coming to a vote. Ending a filibuster requires a vote for cloture, and 60 votes are needed. In addition, the quantity and subjects of amendments are unlimited in the Senate.

Passage of laws usually is required in both the House and Senate. Sometimes identical bills are passed in both chambers. However, often there are differences that need to be resolved by a conference committee with members from the House and Senate. Once the conference committee has agreed upon modified wording, the House and Senate must approve the final bill.

Once a bill is approved by the House and Senate, it requires the signature of the President to become law. The President can sign a bill within the required 10 days (excluding Sundays), making it law. Alternatively, the President may veto the bill. In order to become law, a vetoed bill has to be passed by a two-thirds majority of the House and Senate.

The President's third option is called a pocket veto. A pocket veto can be accomplished if Congress is no longer in session and the President does not sign the bill within the 10-day time limit. In that case, the bill dies.

It is helpful for physicians to understand the political process and to be available to our legislators to assist when important bills are introduced. A sponsor from one district commonly requires support from committee members and subcommittee members from various districts and parties. In some cases, communication to those committee members from their own voting constituents (us) can be a powerful factor in saving a bill from being tabled and dying in committee. It is important for us to understand and exercise our abilities to assist in the legislative process.

The various states have somewhat similar processes. Physicians are encouraged to learn about them. Baker and Morse prepared a useful summary of both federal and state processes.1 That article was the primary source for this chapter. Readers who have found this information of interest are encouraged to consult the original article to find similar information about state legislatures, in which approximately 80,000 bills are introduced annually with approximately 23,000 (28.8%) becoming law.1 It is essential that our voices be heard by our legislators and that we remain sufficiently knowledgeable to be able to help well-meaning legislators articulate sensible bills and guide them to becoming law.

References

1. Baker M, Morse S. How a bill becomes a law. *Bull Am Coll Surg* 2008;93(12):26–7, 47.

Reprinted with modifications by permission of Vendome Group from:
Sataloff RT. Establishing federal laws. *ENT J* 2013;92(2):52–6.

43. New problems in the scope-of-practice controversy

Patient safety and quality of care are primary concerns for physicians and all responsible allied health professionals. However, disagreements between physicians and allied health professionals have occurred, such as between otolaryngologists and audiologists, ophthalmologists and optometrists, anesthesiologists and nurse anesthetists, and others. Most allied health professionals recognize and agree that medical diagnosis is not within their scope of practice and that diagnosis requires a physician. Nevertheless, bills appear frequently in state legislatures that contain language such as 'diagnosis' within the scope of practice of audiologists and speech pathologists. Similar scope-of-practice concerns have arisen around the endoscopic diagnosis of voice and swallowing disorders, laser surgery by optometrists (who are not physicians) and others.

In general, the discussions and debates have been vigorous but civil, and relationships between most physicians and most allied health professionals remain good, as do relations between our professional organizations for the most part, despite some disagreements over scope of practice.

As an example of collaboration, a development has introduced a potential patient risk about which physicians and audiologists are united in steadfast agreement. In many jurisdictions, hearing aids cannot be sold without a purchaser either having a medical evaluation and hearing health diagnosis, or signing a waiver declining medical consultation. This process was intended to protect the general public from inappropriate hearing aid sales and to prevent delayed diagnosis of serious conditions. However, the process was undermined and bypassed by UnitedHealth Group (UHG), the company that offers health insurance and other services through United-Healthcare (UHC).

By revenue, UHC is the largest health insurer in the United States. On October 3, 2011, UHC announced that it would provide its clients and the general public with online hearing testing and, on the basis of those hearing tests, would permit the purchase of hearing aids through the Internet, operating through HealthInnovations (HHI), a subsidiary company of UHG. HHI contracted IntriCon Corporation (Arden Hills, Minn.) to manufacture its hearing aids.

Most reputable hearing aid manufacturers have a public policy against the sale of their hearing aids online. Therefore, the HHI model was in conflict with the standard of practice within the hearing aid industry. This is no small issue. Even if this policy involved only UHG/UHC's clients and not the general public, the impact would be substantial. UHG/UHC clearly established an aggressive strategy targeting the elderly population. Also on October 3, 2011, UHC introduced a new Medicare plan and began marketing actively to the elderly. The company has the financial and organizational ability to reach a great many people. However, the decision to offer online diagnosis, treatment, and hearing aid distribution for hearing-impaired patients raised major concerns among otolaryngologists and audiologists.

On October 31, 2011, the Academy of Doctors of Audiology and the American Academy of Audiology sent a joint letter to UHC expressing their concerns.1 Otolaryngologists share those concerns. An online evaluation is no substitute for a thorough examination by an otolaryngologist with comprehensive audiometry performed by a certified audiologist, followed by appropriate testing leading to an accurate diagnosis of hearing impairment. It will not be surprising if the online testing and hearing aid dispensing process leads to delayed diagnosis of serious and potentially treatable conditions.

It is not clear whether UHG/UHC will be liable for missed or incorrect diagnoses or whether, in its role as an insurance company, it will have legislative immunity (under the Employee Retirement Income Security Act (ERISA)). One might argue that such protection would not be appropriate since the insurance company is clearly venturing into the practice of medicine with this initiative. However, one might make the same argument about insurance company 'medical directors' who determine what studies and operations our patients may or may not have (the practice of medicine, it seems to me); and yet the insurance companies generally enjoy protection from the consequences of their actions, when similar actions by individual practitioners could result in malpractice suits.

This new approach by UHG/UHC was considered a matter for serious investigation in and of itself, and it was feared that it marked the beginning of a new trend in the delivery of hearing health and/or geriatric care, which was even more disturbing. Not surprisingly, this beginning has lead to policies that are likely to be worse. Before long, hearing aids are likely to be available over the counter with no physician or allied health involvement. Physicians and legislatures need to monitor the consequences of such changes closely with particular attention to delayed diagnosis of potentially treatable and sometimes serious disorders.

References

1. The Academy of Doctors of Audiology. The Academy of Doctors of Audiology warns consumers against obtaining hearing aids without proper diagnosis, treatment and counseling. November 22, 2011. https://www.audiologyonline.com/releases/academy-doctors-audiology-warns-consumers-2048. Accessed September 20, 2018.

Reprinted with modifications by permission of Vendome Group from:

Sataloff RT. New problems in the scope-of-practice controversy. *ENT J* 2012;91(3):92–5.

Part V: Clinical Practice

44. Was that my doctor?

Confusion among patients about what kind of healthcare provider they have seen is pervasive. While reputable professionals in all disciplines are responsible about avoiding confusion and potential adverse health consequences, problems still exist. Ophthalmologists have extensive experience with this issue. Many patients have seen optometrists who accurately identify themselves as 'doctor', and such patients often believe incorrectly that they have seen an ophthalmologist and had a comprehensive, medical diagnostic eye examination. Recently, a growing number of optometrists would argue that they have. Optometrists have been attempting to expand their scope of practice to include diagnosis and treatment, including laser surgery, and these attempts have been successful in some states.

Patients with otolaryngologic disorders have encountered similar problems. This is particularly disturbing to many of us when these problems involve elderly patients. In some cases, the problems have been created by hearing aid dealers with little beyond a high school education, who wear white coats and do not correct patients who address them as 'doctor'. These hearing aid sales people look in patients' ears, have them sign forms, including the one declining referral for a medical examination, and sell them hearing aids. Many of these patients believe that they have seen an ear doctor.

It should be noted that the associations of hearing aid dealers and their reputable members are as troubled by such behavior as are otolaryngologists, but it still occurs. The problem has gotten worse recently with the increasing number of audiologists who have Doctor of Audiology (AuD) degrees and can properly refer to themselves as 'doctor'. The vast majority of audiologists are entirely reputable and meticulous about informing their patients of who and what they are, and they are not exceeding their scope of practice. However, there are troublesome exceptions, particularly among

AuD audiologists with independent hearing aid businesses who allow their patients to think that their visit with the audiologist constitutes having seen an ear doctor.

In Pennsylvania, the problem reached such proportion that a law was passed to address it. Other states are taking or contemplating similar actions. The Pennsylvania law imposed some minor inconveniences, but they have been overshadowed by the intent and benefit of the legislation.

The Pennsylvania law was signed on November 23, 2010, and was intended to ensure that patients would not be deceived by health professionals who misrepresent their training. The law was designed to make sure patients know who is taking care of them. Under the new law, all healthcare providers are required to wear photo identification badges that state their credentials in large block letters. These will include descriptions such as 'registered nurse' or 'physician'.

All healthcare employers were required to comply, effective June 2015. Compliance still is not perfect. However, it is important for all of us to recognize that the problem exists and to seek solutions in our own jurisdictions.

The Pennsylvania legislation is certainly not the only approach, but it is comforting to note that the problem has been recognized to be of magnitude sufficient to warrant legislative intervention. Physicians in all specialties should be proactive with local and state leaders in helping to ensure patient safety through identification of inappropriate conduct and development of effective remedies.

Reprinted with modifications by permission of Vendome Groupe from:
Sataloff RT. Was that my doctor? *ENT J* 2011;90(12):562.

45. Women in Otolaryngology–Head and Neck Surgery

Women are now well established in medicine, but historically this was not always true. Hence, it seems reasonable for each specialty to analyze itself from time to time to determine where it stands on the inclusion of women in practice and in leadership positions. While otolaryngology–head and neck surgery has generally been considered a woman-friendly surgical subspecialty, we, too, should assess our field to be certain that we are doing as well as we might think we are.

In 2015, the Association of American Medical Colleges (AAMC) reported that nearly 39% of physicians in the United States were women; 47.9% of accepted medical school applicants and 46.3% of graduating medical students were women.[1] Those figures represent substantial progress. For example, only 9% of accepted applicants and 7% of graduates in 1965 were female.[1] As of July 2010, 1,346 women in otolaryngology were active members of the American Academy of Otolaryngology–Head and Neck Surgery (AAO–HNS), representing 12.4% of the membership.[2] As of March 2011, 1,724 out of 11,868 (14.5%) members of the AAO–HNS were women (with 220 members unidentified by gender).[3] Currently, of the 12,000 members of the AAO-HNS, about 2,200 are women.[4]

AAMC data show that about two-thirds of women physicians practice in six specialties.[1] One is anesthesiology; the other five rank among the lowest-paying specialties in medicine (family practice (54.5%), internal medicine (43.2%), obstetrics and gynecology (82.8%), pediatrics (71.7%), and psychiatry (54.1%)). The reasons for this disproportionate distribution are uncertain. While some of these fields have shorter residencies (if fellowships are excluded) than some of the surgical fields, the old argument about better lifestyles is certainly open to challenge, as anyone who has taken call in obstetrics or pediatrics knows well.

Additional AAMC data indicate that women have been pursuing residencies in other fields with increasing frequency: In 2015, 25.6% of urology residents were been women, as were 66.7% in allergy and immunology, 62.9% in dermatology, about 37% in colon and rectal surgery, 65.6% in medical genetics, 48.4% in neurology, 42.6% in ophthalmology, 36.1% in otolaryngology, 52% in pathology, 46% in preventive medicine, and 38.2% in general surgery.[1]

I made multiple attempts to determine what percentage of applicants to otolaryngology residency programs are women and what percentage of accepted residents are women, but this information is not available through AAO–HNS, the American Board of Otolaryngology, the Association of Academic Departments of Otolaryngology–Head and Neck Surgery, the National Resident Matching Program (NRMP), or numerous other sources.

Women surgeons have taken various approaches to involvement in organized medicine. The board of directors of AAO–HNS established a section on Women in Otolaryngology (WIO). Interestingly, female otolaryngologists organized their efforts within the Academy rather than separately. This made Otolaryngology–HNS the first surgical subspecialty that did not have a women's organization established outside the subspecialty's academy, rather than within the traditional organization. WIO is a valuable influence within the AAO-HNS and the field of otolaryngology.

In the United States of America, women have become more prominent in leadership positions in the past decade. According to the AAMC, between 2003 and 2008, the number of women associates and vice-chairs increased by 73% (all fields of medicine), and the number of women division chiefs more than doubled.[5] As of 2015, 20.5% of permanent medical school basic science chairs and 13.7% of clinical chairs were women.[1] There were female deans at 16 U.S. medical schools (12%).[5] In 2015, 16% of permanent deans were women. The first woman medical school dean in the United States was Ann Preston, M.D. who founded Women's Medical College and became its dean in 1866. Leah Lowenstein, who was appointed to the position at Jefferson Medical College, Thomas Jefferson University, in 1982, was the first female dean at another medical school in the U.S.

I surveyed many of the major otolaryngology journals to determine the number of women who serve as their editors and on their editorial boards. Of all the journals surveyed, none has a female Editor-in-Chief.

The number of women, total number of members, and percentages of women on editorial boards are as follows:

- *American Journal of Otolaryngology–Head and Neck Medicine and Surgery*: 5 of 44 (11.4%)
- *American Journal of Rhinology & Allergy*: 9 of 51 (17.6%)
- *Annals of Otology, Rhinology & Laryngology*: 7 of 61 (11.5%)
- *Archives of Otolaryngology–Head & Neck Surgery*: 5 of 17 (29.4%)
- *Ear, Nose & Throat Journal*: 24 of 154 (15.6%)
- *Head & Neck*: 10 of 63 (15.9%)
- *Journal of the Association for Research in Otolaryngology*: 11 of 26 (42.3%)
- *The Journal of Laryngology and Otology*: 3 of 42 (7.1%)
- *The Journal of Otolaryngology–Head & Neck Surgery*: 4 of 25 (16%)
- *Journal of Vestibular Research*: 2 of 14 (14.3%)
- *Journal of Voice*: 57 of 126 (45.2%)
- *The Laryngoscope*: 10 of 86 (11.6%)
- *Operative Techniques in Otolaryngology–Head and Neck Surgery*: 2 of 23 (8.7%)
- *Otolaryngology–Head and Neck Surgery*: 12 of 39 (30.8%)
- *Otology & Neurotology*: 23 of 168 (13.7%)

Despite these advances, there are still discrepancies between male and female medical professionals. One important issue is reimbursement. For example, Lo Sasso et al. evaluated New York data from 1999 through 2008 and discovered that newly trained male residents earned a mean of $16,819 more than female physicians in 2008, compared with a difference of $3,600 in 1999.[6] The gender gap extended across specialties, practice types, and locations. According to the authors, it could not be explained by the number of hours worked. The problem has continued. For example, the most recent data (2017) show full-time male otolaryngologists earn 7% more than females ($401,000 vs. $375,000).[7]

Having read the literature, I am unable to discern a reason for the gender gap in compensation in our field, or in other fields. It has been suggested that 'female physicians may be seeking out employment arrangements that compensate them in other, nonfinancial ways, and more employers may be beginning to offer such arrangements'.[6]

While it is possible (as has been speculated) that women are earning less money by choice in order to have more flexible lifestyles, minimize unpredictable weekend on-call commitments, etc., I am not aware of any data confirming those speculations. I believe that it is dangerous for us to make that assumption. Along with the rest of medicine, otolaryngology should study this important issue to be certain that gender bias has been eliminated from our specialty.

References

1. American Association of Medical Colleges. The State of Women in Academic Medicine: The Pipeline and Pathways to Leadership, 2015–2016. https://www.aamc.org/members/gwims/statistics/. Accessed September 23, 2018.
2. Malekzadeh S. Women in Otolaryngology Committee. *AAO–HNS Bulletin*. July 2010, p. 48.
3. Personal communication. Lani Cadow, AAO–HNS. March 22, 2011.
4. American Association of Medical Colleges. Women in U.S. academic medicine statistics and benchmarking, 2009–2010. http://www.aamc.org/members/gwims/statistics/. Accessed July 14, 2011.
5. Personal communication. AAO-HNS. September 24, 2018.
6. Lo Sasso AT, Richards MR, Chou CF, Gerber SE. The $16,819 pay gap for newly trained physicians: The unexplained trend of men earning more than women. *Health Aff (Millwood)* 2011;30(2):193–201.
7. Grisham S. Medscape Otolaryngologist Compensation Report 2017. April 12, 2017. https://www.medscape.com/slideshow/compensation-2017-otolaryngology-6008581#8. Accessed September 28, 2018.

Reprinted with modifications by permission of Vendome Group from:
Sataloff RT. Women in otolaryngology–head and neck surgery. *ENT J* 2011;90(8):330–2

46. Disruptive physicians: Sound more familiar than you thought?

Over the course of a career, many physicians serve in leadership positions, such as chair of a department in a university of hospital or clinical service chief. In such roles, we are called upon routinely to address a variety of problems with important ethical and legal ramifications about which we have received little or no training during residency. Disruptive physician behavior is one of such problems. Not only are most doctors unaware of the subtleties and literature regarding this topic, but most of us also are unfamiliar with the current definition of disruptive behavior.

In today's 'politically correct' environment, an intuitive impression of what constitutes disruptive behavior might not be an adequate definition for any of us, but especially for those physicians in leadership positions, particularly when a complaint is lodged. We are already familiar with changes in definition that have evolved over the past few decades. For example, comments that many of us have considered innocent, good-natured banter (or even outright compliments) are now grounds for sexual harassment actions. Similarly, disruptive physician behavior might include activities that many of us regard as 'temperamental' but that we might not recognize as potentially actionable.

The American Medical Association (AMA) has written, 'Personal conduct, whether verbal or physical, that affects or that potentially may affect patient care negatively constitutes disruptive behavior. (This includes but is not limited to conduct that interferes with one's ability to work with other members of the health care team.)"[1]

Under this definition, some behaviors would be recognized by all of us as disruptive, but others might not. For example, obviously disruptive behaviors include failure to carry out medical responsibilities, such as failing to answer pages when on call or to respond to requests by other healthcare workers to assist in patient care; sexually inappropriate behavior; use of racially inappropriate language and use of foul language (commonly defined by the listener).

Less obvious disruptive behaviors include displays of anger deemed inappropriate by other members of the medical staff that could be seen as intimidating to coworkers. This may include yelling or in other ways chastising operating room staff for what the surgeon perceives as performance error or inefficiency. Such allegations do not require the presence of patient harm, physical intimidation, sexual harassment, or negative physician intent. In fact, physicians typically consider their behavior as reasonable and appropriate to the situation. Many surgeons consider it appropriate and even desirable to be fairly demanding in the operating room, and our behavior might not be different from that of some of the better (but temperamental) surgeons who trained us. However, in this politically correct world, such behavior may be challenged by nursing and anesthesia staff as disruptive, particularly when it is habitual and striking enough to cause some members of the staff to request that they not be assigned to work with us.

In past years, many of us considered this acceptable operating room behavior and potentially beneficial because it helped weed out of our team people with whom we really did not want to work and select for ourselves the 'best' nurses most suited to our surgical care. Today, however, such 'normal' operating room interaction can result in complaints of disruptive behavior that cannot be ignored by hospitals.

The Health Care Quality Improvement Act, passed in 1986, not only created the National Practitioner Data Bank (NPDB), but it also designated reporting and oversight responsibilities for physicians to a variety of healthcare agencies and committees.[2] Subsequently, the AMA recommended that each medical staff develop bylaws 'for intervening in situations where a physician's behavior is identified as disruptive'.[1] The Joint Commission also requires that hospitals develop policies regarding disruptive physicians.[3] Hence, hospitals are required to investigate and address complaints of disruptive behavior in a formal and judicious manner. In some cases, the evaluation includes agencies outside the hospital, such as the state medical society; and some physician misconduct must be reported to the state medical board and the NPDB.

Some hospitals employ the consultative services of a forensic psychiatrist as part the investigation/evaluation process. The forensic psychiatrist evaluates the complaint and may recommend that the accused physician undergo psychiatric treatment and workplace oversight. Physicians (particularly those in leadership positions) might benefit from reading reviews of this topic by Meyer and Price,[4] and by Santin and Kaups.[5]

The politically correct culture of the late 20th and early 21st century has had a substantial impact on interpersonal interaction and humor. Although some of us find many of its consequences objectionable, political correctness has created new standards that have substantial legal and professional implications that affect all of us in our dealings with colleagues, coworkers, and patients. It is important for physicians to be familiar with evolving definitions and concepts of acceptable behavior and with the obligations, rights, processes, and protections available when allegations of disruptive behavior are raised. Familiarity with the most current concepts is advisable for all physicians; and it is essential for any physician in a leadership role, such as department chair, service chief, or representative to the executive committee of a hospital medical staff.

References

1. American Medical Association. Opinions on professional rights and responsibilities. Physicians with disruptive behavior. Opinion E-9.045. Adopted June 2000. Available at http://www.ama-assn.org/ama/pub/category/8533.html/. Last accessed Feb. 4, 2008.
2. The Health Care Quality Improvement Act of 1986, as amended 42 USC 11101 1/26/98. Available at http://www.npdb-hipdb.hrsa.gov/legislation/title4.html/. Last accessed Feb. 4, 2008.
3. Youssi MD. JCAHO standards help address disruptive physician behavior. *Physician Exec* 2002;28(6):12–3.
4. Meyer DJ, Price M. Forensic psychiatric assessments of behaviorally disruptive physicians. *J Am Acad Psychiatry Law* 2006;34(1):72–81.
5. Santin BJ, Kaups KL. The disruptive physician: Addressing the issues. *Bull Am Coll Surg* 2015;100(2):20–4.

Reprinted with modifications by permission of Vendome Group from:
Sataloff RT. Disruptive physicians: Sound more familiar than you thought? *ENT J* 2008;87(3):124–7.

47. Hearing loss: Economic impact

More and more of us are living long enough to experience hearing loss. According to the National Institute on Deafness and Other Communication Disorders (NIDCD), as of December 15, 2016, approximately 37.5 million American adults (about 15%) report having some degree of hearing loss.[1] There is a strong correlation between hearing loss and age. 8.5% of Americans between 55 and 64 years of age, nearly 25% between 65 and 74, and 50% 75 years or older have impaired hearing.[1]

The NIDCD estimates also that 28.8 million people who could benefit from a hearing aid. As an added annoyance, roughly 25 million Americans have experienced tinnitus.[1] Most otolaryngologists are familiar with the inconveniences associated with hearing impairment. Its adverse effect on quality of life has been recognized for decades. However, somewhat less attention has been paid to the effects of hearing impairment on earning power. While additional evidence-based studies would be helpful, interesting data are reported through the Better Hearing Institute (BHI). An article on that site revealed that untreated hearing loss can decrease a household's income by as much as $12,000 per year and that use of amplification mitigates that effect by 50%.[2] Despite the need for confirmation of this claim, a relationship between hearing loss and income seems credible.

Employees who have difficulty hearing supervisors, instructions, and customers are unlikely to perform as well as their coworkers with normal hearing. Mistakes made because of misunderstanding verbal instruction not only impair employment, but they also are likely to be associated with increased job stress as the impaired individual struggles to compensate for hearing loss and avoid making mistakes. As more baby boomers remain in the workforce longer, this problem is likely to increase, and it is important for us to be cognizant of the problem and help prevent losses of jobs and decreases in income associated with remediable hearing loss.

When the problem is considered throughout society rather than individually, the impact becomes more apparent. In calculating their data, the BHI researchers assumed that there are 31 million Americans with hearing loss (rather than the 37.5 million estimated by the NIDCD). The BHI researchers analyzed impact on the 24 million hearing-impaired individuals who do not use amplification and estimated the economic impact to be $100 million. That corresponds with a loss of $18 billion in potential federal taxes, assuming that they are all in the 15% tax bracket.[2]

NIDCD noted that only 20% of patients who will benefit from hearing aids wear them.[1] Moreover, many people with untreated hearing loss have undergone a professional hearing test.

While acknowledging the need to add to the body of literature studying the association between hearing impairment and income loss, and while recognizing that the statistics reported above and in other literature require confirmation to determine the prevalence and magnitude of the problem, it appears as if we as physicians should at least recognize that there is probably an association between hearing impairment and job performance/ income. Consequently, we should be doing everything possible to help lessen the burden of hearing impairment on our patients and society.

Most of us probably think we already are doing everything possible, but it might be worth reassessing that assumption. One of the striking (if unverified) statistics above is the suggestion that half of the people with hearing impairment have never had an audiogram. This seems believable and is possibly even an underestimate. It is common for us to see even elderly adults who have not had hearing tests since they were school children. Undoubtedly, even some otolaryngologists are contributing to that problem. How often have we seen patients for a specific, non-otologic problem (nasal congestion, chronic cough, etc.) and focused on that problem only, neglecting to inquire about and screen hearing even in high-risk patients such as the elderly?

Admittedly, third-party carriers make this situation worse. If patients do not complain of hearing loss (as is the case with many elderly, hearing impaired patients) and we obtain an audiogram to screen for hearing loss, it is sometimes difficult to get reimbursed, especially if the audiogram is normal. However, this should not discourage us from looking actively and aggressively for unrecognized hearing impairment. Rather, the magnitude of societal costs of the problem should inspire us to develop, promulgate, and follow clinical guidelines for hearing screening in all age groups.

We should consider combining this effort with increased research into the prevalence and societal impact of hearing impairment, as well as with educational programs for the general public and legislators to help increase awareness of the effects of untreated hearing impairment, the importance of comprehensive otologic assessment to identify potentially treatable causes of hearing loss, and the cosmetic and technologic advances in hearing amplification. Such awareness should lead to improvements in quality of life and workplace productivity that will be of great help to the hearing-impaired population, while we are working on the more challenging problems of nerve and hair cell regrowth and hearing restoration.

References

1. National Institute on Deafness and Other Communication Disorders (NIDCD). Quick statistics about hearing. December 15, 2016. https://www.nidcd.nih.gov/health/statistics/quick-statistics-hearing. Accessed September 24, 2018.
2. Kochkin S. The impact of untreated hearing loss on household income. May 2007. Better Hearing Institute. http://www.betterhearing.org/sites/default/files/hearingpedia-resources/M7_Hearing_aids_and_income_2006.pdf. Accessed September 27, 2018.

Reprinted with modifications by permission of Vendome Group from:
  Sataloff RT. Hearing loss: Economic impact. *ENT J* 2012;91(1):10–2.

48. Evaluating occupational hearing loss: The value of the AMA's Guides to the Evaluation of Permanent Impairment

Despite the Occupational Safety and Health Act (OSHA) and other legislation enacted to help prevent occupational hearing loss, noise-induced hearing impairment still occurs. Otolaryngologists are called upon frequently to evaluate claimants who allege that they have suffered work-related hearing impairment. Physicians are involved not only in confirming or refuting the presence of hearing loss, but also in diagnosing its cause and helping to determine the degree to which it might have impacted a person's life or caused disability or handicap.

Fortunately for everyone concerned, physicians do not have to depend on individual experience and unsubstantiated opinion to make such judgments. The medical and scientific community has nationally (and in some cases internationally) accepted standards to guide such judgments so that they can be as valid, reliable, fair, and as consistent as possible across individuals, geographical locations, and even organ systems.

All physicians involved with evaluations of impairment and disability should be familiar with the American Medical Association's (AMA's) *Guides to the Evaluation of Permanent Impairment*[1] in order to be able to comply with the standard of care.

It is important to understand the Guides in historical context in order to appreciate the value of this dynamic book and its importance as a scientific compendium. In the United States, physicians from all specialties have been developing and refining the Guides for more than half a century. The AMA established an ad hoc committee in 1956 that led to a publication in the *Journal of the American Medical Association* (*JAMA*) in 1958 called 'A guide to the evaluation of permanent impairment of the extremities and back'.[2] By 1970, a total of 13 such Guides had appeared in *JAMA*. They were collected as a compendium in 1971 and published as the first edition of the Guides.[3] The value and importance of the Guides became apparent, and great effort has been devoted to revising and improving the book.

In 1981, the AMA established 12 expert panels in preparation for the second edition, which was published in 1984. The third (1988), fourth (1993), fifth (2000), and sixth (2008) editions all contained important changes, many of which are summarized in the introductory chapters of each edition. However, the most striking changes were promulgated throughout the sixth edition, to which I was privileged to contribute as lead author for the otolaryngology chapter.

I had followed the process for many years through my father, Joseph Sataloff, M.D., who was a contributor or chapter editor for otolaryngology for the second through fifth editions. I also serve as the American Academy of Otolaryngology-Head and Neck Surgery's (AAO-HNS) Advisory Committee Representative to the AMA for Evaluation of Permanent Impairment. This chapter reviews some of the valuable perspective gained through these activities. It is hoped that the insights summarized herein will assist clinicians, attorneys and others in understanding the genesis of the Guides, and the importance of their proper application.

As scientific knowledge and methodology expand, and our knowledge base grows, it is essential for physicians and scientists to incorporate new knowledge and allow our practices to evolve. The Guides have been strikingly successful in this regard, especially the most recent edition. It warrants discussion because it has some fundamental differences from the first five editions, with which all physicians should be familiar. Each new edition has incorporated the latest scientific research and practice.

The first five editions provided the best available information for evaluating permanent impairment, but they had some shortcomings that were acknowledged by most of the scientific community, including by those involved in writing the Guides. The sixth edition incorporates a radical paradigm shift to a simplified, function-based, internally consistent model of disablement that has rectified many of the concerns about earlier editions. The new approach involves using the internationally accepted International Classification of Functioning, Disability and Health (ICF).[4] The latest edition of the Guides also focuses more directly on diagnosis, using evidence-based medicine when possible; simplicity to optimize inter-rater and intra-rater reliability; functionally based ratings percentages; and consistent conceptual and methodologic approaches and ratings across organ systems.

The ICF model is a comprehensive classification for describing and measuring health and disability in individuals and populations. It assesses bodily functions and structures (including impairments), activity (including activity limitations), and participation in life situations (including participation restrictions). It relates the health condition of an individual to environmental and personal factors. This internationally accepted approach represents a major improvement toward which contributors to the Guides have been striving for many years. Developing the ICF model was a complex process, and it was not complete by the time the fifth edition was printed.

The ICF arose from a worldwide consensus process, was endorsed by the World Health Assembly in 2001,[5] and has been accepted as a member of the World Health Organization family of international classifications. The AMA's Guides has now adopted ICF terminology and definitions and used this approach to refine evaluation of impairment, disability, and impairment rating. This approach has created greater consistency within and between organ systems and established impairment and disability classifications based on the latest available evidence and expert consensus. Emphasis was placed on precision, accuracy, reliability, and validity. However, evaluation of functional impact was enhanced using the 5-point scale taxonomy created by the ICF. The approach allows incorporation of information from the history, physical findings, objective test results, functional assessment, and, when appropriate, determining the burden of treatment compliance.

The revision process for each chapter in the Guides is not only rigorous, but also multidisciplinary. For example, contributors to the otolaryngology chapter included not only otolaryngologists, but also physicians in other specialties such as occupational and environmental medicine and pulmonology. As an example, all aspects of the otolaryngology chapter were reexamined and researched during the revision process. Literature was searched for new evidence and new consensus opinions, and the content of our chapter was compared with overlapping content in other chapters to optimize consistency across organ systems.

This revision effort included reviewing the formula used for calculating hearing impairment. The original approach to this problem was published in 1959.[6] That formula used 500 Hz, 1,000 Hz, and 2,000 Hz. Based on additional study, the formula was revised to include 3,000 Hz in 1979.[7] Higher frequencies are not included because they are not necessary to understand speech. For example, most early telephones used through the 1960s did not transmit frequencies above 2,800 Hz through their earpieces, and speech comprehension on those devices was not problematic.

Since 1979, considerable conjecture and opinion have been promulgated supporting the formula as it stands[8-14] and advocating changes in the formula[15]; and there has been vast experience in applying it for more than 30 years. After reassessment of available data, the relevant committees of the AAO-HNS, as well as other expert clinicians and the authors of the otolaryngology chapter in the sixth edition of the Guides, have found no credible evidence to support revising the formula again. In addition, the consensus and evidence still indicate that puretone audiometry is the most appropriate test in this population for estimating an individual's ability to hear speech. While other audiometric tests can be used in the diagnostic process, measures such as the discrimination score can be manipulated so easily that they cannot be considered a valid standard for routine determination of hearing performance in medicolegal settings. Consequently, the AAO-HNS formula remains the basis for the formula in the AMA Guides.

As a result of the exceedingly rigorous scientific process through which the Guides was developed and has evolved, the publication has been recognized and accepted nationally. In nearly all U.S. territories, states and commonwealths, the AMA's Guides is either recommended or mandated for use by Workers' Compensation law. It also is used for actions involving the Federal Employees' Compensation Act, Longshore and Harbor Workers' Compensation Act, and Federal Employees' Compensation laws. AMA's *Guides to the Evaluation of Permanent Impairment* is the premier compendium of scientific evidence and expert opinion related to the topic and has been accepted as establishing the standard of care by the AMA and essentially all major specialty societies in the United States.

Physicians involved with patients being assessed for possible work-related impairment should be not only loosely familiar with the Guides from past editions, but also current on the latest scientific and methodologic advances in the most recent edition of this definitive reference.

References

1. American Medical Association. *Guides to the evaluation of permanent impairment.* 6th Ed. Chicago, Illinois: American Medical Association; 2008.
2. American Medical Association. A guide to the evaluation of permanent impairment of the extremities and back. *J Am Med Assoc* 1958; 166 (Special No.): 1–109.

3. Guides to the Evaluation of Permanent Impairment. Chicago, Illinois: American Medical Association; 1971.
4. World Health Organization. International Classification of Functioning, Disability and Health (ICF). Geneva, Switzerland: World Health Organization; 2001.
5. Resolution of the World Health Organization. International classification of functioning, disability and health. 54th World Health Assembly; May 22, 2001.
6. Guide for the evaluation of hearing impairment, a report of the Committee on Conservation of Hearing. *Transactions of the American Academy of Ophthalmology and Otolaryngology* 1959;63(2).
7. American Academy of Otolaryngology Committee on Hearing and Equilibrium and American Council of Otolaryngology Committee on the Medical Aspects of Noise. Guide for the evaluation of hearing handicap. *JAMA* 1979;241(19):2055–9.
8. Dobie RA, Sakai CS. Monetary compensation for hearing loss: Clinician's survey. *J OHL* 1998;1(1):73–80.
9. Doerfler LG, Nett EM, Matthews J. The relationships between audiologic measures and handicap: Part one. *J OHL* 1998;1(2):103–52.
10. Dobie RA, Sakai CS. Monetary compensation for hearing loss: Choice and weighting of frequencies. *J OHL* 1998;1(3):163–71.
11. Doerfler LG, Nett EM, Matthews J. The relationships between audiologic measures and handicap: Part two. *J OHL* 1998;1(3):213–35.
12. Sataloff J, Vassallo LA, Sataloff RT. The validity of the AMA impairment formula for hearing loss. *J OHL* 1998;1(4):237–42.
13. Doerfler LG, Nett EM, Matthews J. The relationships between audiologic measures and handicap: Part 3. *J OHL* 1998;1(4):243–64.
14. Nelson RA. Development of the AMA formula or who built this camel anyway? *Journal of Occupational Hearing Loss* 1999;2(4):145–51.
15. American Speech-Language-Hearing Association Task Force on the Definition of Hearing Handicap. On the definition of hearing handicap. https://www.asha.org/policy/rp1981-00022.htm. Accessed September 24, 2018.

Reprinted with modifications by permission of Vendome Group from:
    Sataloff RT. Evaluating occupational hearing loss: The value of the AMA's Guides to the Evaluation of Permanent Impairment. *ENT J* 2014;93(4-5):132–5.

49. Emotional intelligence and physician wellness

Emotional intelligence (EI) is the ability to recognize and manage one's own emotions and the emotions of other people.[1] It involves the ability to be aware of one's own emotions, the ability to control emotions and apply them to various tasks including problem solving and thinking, and the ability to manage emotions including regulating one's own emotions, and affecting the emotions of other people (e.g. cheering them up or calming them down). Intuitively, many of us recognize high EI as beneficial, but there are relatively few data confirming this intuition. One good study investigated the relationship between EI and resident well-being.[2] While the investigators did not gather data on practicing physicians, it is reasonable to speculate that they might be similar.

Various aspects of resident well-being have been studied more extensively than the well-being of practitioners. Among surgical residents, for example, a burnout rate of 60.3% has been identified, along with emotional exhaustion and depersonalization.[2] Depression rates among residents and practicing physicians have been reported from 22% to 50%.[3-5] Moreover, it has been established that the risk of suicide in male residents is 1.5 to 3.8 fold greater than age-matched and sex-matched peers in the general population, and the successful suicide rate for female residents is 3.7 to 4.5 fold higher.[6,7]

Lin et al. studied surgical residents in a single program.[2] They measured emotional intelligence with the Trait Emotional Intelligence Questionnaire-Short Form; and they used the Dupuy Psychological General Well-Being Index, the Maslach

Burnout Inventory and Beck Depression Inventory Short Form to evaluate resident wellness. Correlations provided very interesting insights. Emotional intelligence was found to be a strong predictor of residents' well-being. Residents with high EI did better in residency than those with lower EI scores. High EI scores correlated with psychological well-being. They also correlated inversely with depression, emotional exhaustion, depersonalization and two parameters of burnout.

The study by Lin et al. not only provided these observations but also confirmed the high prevalence of burnout and depression among surgical residents. 82% of the residents responding met criteria for burnout, and the emotional exhaustion and depersonalization scores were disturbingly high. These numbers were higher than the reported burnout rates for surgeons in practice (28% to 48%).[4,6] This suggests that some of the adverse factors affecting physician wellness might change with circumstance. It is also possible that they can be changed with interventions that increase EI. Since it seems clear that approximately 1/3 to 1/2 of surgical residents meet criteria for depression, and since resident suicides continue to occur (as do suicides among practicing physicians), it seems appropriate for us to be concerned about all factors that might predict emotional difficulties, and to seek information on all interventions that might mitigate them. In Lin's study, EI was the only significant predictor of burnout, depression and psychological well-being.[2]

Emotional intelligence is associated with 'noncognitive attributes that help individuals perceive and regulate emotions and in turn, cope effectively with emotive situations, such as environmental stressors or interpersonal relationships.'[2] It is a significant predictor of physical and mental health in numerous populations. It has been shown to protect individuals against mental health abnormalities including depression and burnout.[8-11]

For physicians, when we interview potential residents, associates, or perhaps even physician extenders and nurses, we tend to rely on interview impressions and previous past performance. Perhaps it is time for us to research whether EI is as important among physicians in other fields and non-physicians as it is among general surgeons and to consider subjective and formal evaluations of EI in our selection process.

References

1. Salovey P, Mayer JD. Emotional Intelligence. *Imagin Cogn Pers* 1990;185–211.
2. Lin D, Liebert CA, Tran J, et al. Emotional Intelligence as a Predictor of Resident Well-Being. *JACS* 2016;223(2):352–8.

3. Dyrbye LN, West CP, Satele D, et al. Burnout among US medical students, residents, and early career physicians relative to the general US population. *Acad Med* 2014;89:443–51.
4. Shanafelt TD, Balch CM, Bechamps GJ, et al. Burnout and career satisfaction among American surgeons. *Ann Surg* 2009;250:463–71.
5. Collier VU, McCue JD, Markus A, Smith L. Stress in medical residency: status quo after a decade of reform? *Ann Intern Med* 2002;136:384–90.
6. Balch CM, Freischlag JA, Shanafelt TD. Stress and burnout among surgeons: understanding and managing the syndrome and avoiding the adverse consequences. *Arch Surg* 2009;144:371–6.
7. Schernhammer ES, Colditz GA. Suicide rates among physicians: a quantitative and gender assessment (meta-analysis). *Am J Psychiatry* 2004;161:2295–302.
8. Oginska-Bulik N. Emotional intelligence in the workplace: exploring its effects on occupational stress and health outcomes in human service workers. *Int J Occup Med Enviro Health* 2005;18:167–75.
9. Mavroveli S, Petrides KV, Rieffe C, Bakker F. Trait emotional intelligence, psychological well-being and peer-rated social competence in adolescence. *Br J Dev Psychol* 2007;25:263–75.
10. Mikolajczak J, Petrides KV, Hurry J. Adolescents choosing self-harm as an emotion regulation strategy: the protective role of trait emotional intelligence. *Br J Dev Psychol* 2009;48:181–93.
11. Moon TW, Hur WM. Emotional intelligence, emotional exhaustion, and job performance. *Soc Behav Personal* 2011;39:1087–96.

Reprinted with modifications by permission of Vendome Group from:
Sataloff RT. Emotional Intelligence and Physician Wellness. ENT J, in press.

50. Shoulder injuries related to vaccine administration (SIRVA): A potential problem for all physicians

Are shoulder injuries a problem for physicians in all specialties? If they are caused by treatment in our offices, then the answer is 'yes'. If we have any question about that, plaintiff attorneys will help answer it.

Shoulder injury related to vaccine administration (SIRVA) seem to be a relatively new problem, although the *Washington Post* reported that the CDC has recorded at least 1,200 complaints since 1990.[1] The injuries are caused by injection too high on the arm, and the injected material does not have to be a vaccine. Other materials might cause a problem if they are injected into the wrong place. There is speculation that the prevalence of SIRVA has increased in recent years because so many injections are being given in pharmacies, shopping centers and other non-traditional venues for medical care by personnel who might not have been trained fully in the complex anatomy of the shoulder. Moreover, some of these settings do not provide complete privacy. Consequently, many people loosen their collar and pull down a shirt or blouse exposing only the top of the deltoid, rather than removing clothing as they might do in a private examination room. If they expose only the top of the deltoid, a provider who is not familiar with SIRVA could easily inject the wrong location. It is possible that there are otolaryngologic nurses and medical assistants, and probably also physicians, who are not sufficiently familiar with the potential hazards.

Injections in the arm should not be delivered in the top third of the deltoid muscle. When injections are delivered high in the shoulder, the injected material can penetrate the bursa or rotator cuff. Injections lower into the middle portion of the muscle generally avoid this problem. When the injection ends up too high and deep, SIRVA may develop. Typically, the condition can include chronic shoulder pain, limitation in range of motion, rotator cuff tear, frozen shoulder and nerve damage. SIRVA symptoms may last for months, or they may be permanent. SIRVA can prevent patients from lifting an arm to comb or brush hair, raising an arm above shoulder height, dressing without pain, lifting, and performing other similar activities.

Although this condition is associated classically with vaccination, it is possible for it to occur from injection of other substances. Vaccines commonly are inactivated (made of killed viruses), but they contain substances included to provoke a robust immune response. They are designed to be given in the middle of the deltoid, the portion with the greatest muscle mass. When delivered into the bursa or elsewhere in the joint, the inflammation caused may persist. While it is unlikely that a similar reaction would be seen after the injection of a corticosteroid, it is not inconceivable that similar shoulder problems could occur after injection of an antibiotic, pain medicine, antiemetic, cytotoxic drug or other material that might be injected in a physician's office.

SIRVA was recognized as such an important problem that a federal court was established to adjudicate SIRVA claims. Between 2011 and 2014, the program received 136 claims for SIRVA and awarded compensation for 102 of them, with compensation payments totaling about $16 million.[1]

Although we do not typically think of shoulder injuries as problems associated with most physicians, they certainly will be if we cause them. All physicians and ancillary staff should be familiar with SIRVA, the normal anatomy of the shoulder, and the recommended position in the deltoid muscle for injected materials.

References

1. Cimons M. 'I got a pneumonia shot – and then the pain began.' *Washington Post Health & Science*, October 26, 2015. https://www.washingtonpost.

com/national/health-science/i-got-a-pneumonia-shot--and-then-the-pain-began/2015/10/26/3e465a44-691e-11e5-9ef3-fde182507eac_story.html?utm_term=.2df7c2013d67. Accessed on May 12, 2016.

Acknowledgement

Thanks to Thomas Gowen, JD, for bringing this important topic to my attention.

Reprinted with modifications by permission of Vendome Group from:
Sataloff RT. Shoulder Injuries Related to Vaccine Administration (SIRVA): An ENT Problem? *ENT J*, in press.

51. Part-time physicians

It is generally agreed that our society will experience a shortage of physicians in the workforce over the next few decades.[1] Developing strategies to address this worsening problem is challenging for many reasons, including the validity of assumptions about physician work activities. For example, it does not appear valid to assume that one retiring physician can be replaced by one new physician. The lifestyle preferences and quality-of-life choices of physicians in generation X and generation Y suggest that younger physicians will choose to work fewer hours.

It has been estimated that 1.3 full-time equivalents (FTEs) will be required to replace 1 FTE of physicians of the baby boomer generation.[2] Various approaches to this problem have been proposed, including increasing use of physician extenders (physician assistants and nurse practitioners), increasing the number of trainees, retaining physicians in the workforce longer, and other approaches. The use of physician extenders has already proven helpful in some areas, but the impact of physician extenders may be somewhat less in surgical specialties than it is in primary care specialties.

Increasing the number of funded trainees in the United States would require an amendment to the Balanced Budget Act of 1997. Although the number of medical schools and number of American medical graduates have increased, so far, the government has shown no indication that it will increase the number of postgraduate training positions. Retaining physicians in the workforce for a longer period of time may be a particularly effective solution. Otolaryngology provides an example of relevant concerns for one specialty that can be generalized to all fields.

As otolaryngologists age, many do not wish to continue working 50 or 60 hours per week. However, part-time employment can be an attractive alternative to not working at all. In many surgical specialties, this option has not been readily available. For example, there are relatively few part-time heart surgeons. Otolaryngology has been more accepting than many surgical fields of part-time employment of older physicians who wish to slow down but who are not ready to leave the workforce. Although this transition poses business challenges and has not always been possible, otolaryngologists have used it in many private practice settings, and sometimes even in academic employment models. However, more often, when physicians in many fields including otolaryngology complete their fulltime, active careers, they retire.

Even those otolaryngologists who attempt to remain active part-time as teachers (particularly in academic institutions) often find maintaining supported positions over many years challenging. As of 2011, in academic settings there were 21,200 part-time clinical faculty and 1,950 part-time basic science faculty working in the 126 U.S. medical schools.[3] Pollart et al. predicted in 2014 that these numbers would remain fairly stable.[4] It always has been unfortunate that there are so few opportunities for part-time employment, especially for physicians approaching the end of their careers. Our older, wiser, and more experienced physicians end up leaving the workforce sooner than necessary, depriving younger physicians, residents and students of their wisdom and their firsthand understanding of the history of medicine.

Understanding the looming physician shortage, we need to be concerned about losing these physicians also because of their potential to ameliorate the physician shortage in a particularly effective way (retention of skilled, experienced, expert doctors). Recent research has shown the potential importance of fostering an efficient part-time employment model for otolaryngologists and other surgeons.[4]

Satiani et al. have estimated that the shortage of otolaryngologists in the United States was 838 in 2010.[5] By 2020, it is projected to reach 1,662; by 2030, it will be 2,516; by 2040, it will be 3,387; and by 2050, it will be 4,272.[5] In a survey of physicians (all specialties) ages 50 to 65, 14% planned to retire, but 12% expressed an interest in working part-time, defined as approximately 20 hours per week.[6] This is a fairly realistic number of hours.

Erikson studied physicians older than 50 years working part-time and determined that female physicians work an average of 21.3 hours per week, and male physicians work an average of 16.6 hours per week.[7] Moreover, the number of physicians working part-time has increased. It was 13% in 2005, and up to 19% in 2007.[8] In 2015 and 2016, 12% of male physicians and 25% of female physicians worked part-time.[9] More than half of full-time physicians over 50 years of age have expressed interest in changing to part-time work, and 42.6% have reported that the availability of part-time work would affect their decision to remain active past retirement age.[7]

Presently, about two-thirds of physicians over age 50 are practicing actively.[7] That means approximately one-third have left clinical practice; and this population should be targeted for retention. Offering flexible, part-time employment to this group would be a reasonable strategy to try to keep them in the workforce or return them to clinical activity.

In order to enhance the quality and quantity of physicians in the workforce over the next few decades, it seems advisable for all specialties to investigate ways to become even more 'friendly' to part-time physicians. Private practices and academic departments benefit from the experience and clinical skills of older physicians. It is an advantage to medicine and the general public to facilitate part-time employment of older physicians (and of younger physicians) who do not wish to work full-time, a routine 'norm' within the culture of most specialties. Welcoming an increasing percentage of part-time physicians will potentially enrich the lives of not only the part time physicians, but also the full-time physicians with whom they are associated, and especially the lives of their patients.

References

1. Association of American Medical Colleges. GME Funding and Its Role in Addressing the Physician Shortage. May 29, 2018. https://news.aamc.org/for-the-media/article/gme-funding-doctor-shortage/. Accessed September 22, 2018.
2. Weiss GG. Productivity takes a dip. *Med Econ* 2005;82(22):86–94.
3. Bunton SA, Henderson MK. Handbook of Academic Medicine: How Medical School and Teaching Hospitals Work. Washington, DC: Association of American Medical Colleges; 2013.
4. Pollart SM, Dandar V, Brubaker L, et al. Characteristics, satisfaction, and engagement of part-time faculty at U.S. medical schools. *Acad Med* 2015;90(3):355–64.
5. Satiani B, Williams TE, Ellison EC. The impact of employment of part-time surgeons on the expected surgeon shortage. *J Am Coll Surg* 2011;213(3):345–51.
6. Merritt Hawkins & Associates. 2007 Survey of physicians 50 to 65 years old. http://www.merritthawkins.com/pdf/mha2007olderdocsurvey.pdf. Accessed November 1, 2012.
7. Erikson C. Association of American Medical Colleges. The complexities of physician supply and demand: Projections through 2025. https://members.

aamc. org/eweb/upload/The%20Complexities%20of%20Physician%20Supply.pdf. Accessed November 8, 2012.
8. Elliott VS. Making part time work. American Medical News. September 26, 2011. http://www.ama-assn.org/amednews/2011/09/26/bisa0926.htm. Accessed November 8, 2012.
9. Peckham C. Medscape Physician Compensation Report 2016. April 1, 2016. https://www.medscape.com/features/slideshow/compensation/2016/public/overview. Accessed September 27, 2018.

Reprinted with modifications by permission of Vendome Group from:
Sataloff RT. Part-time otolaryngologists. *ENT J* 2012;91(12):512–4.

52. Adverse surgical events: Effects on the surgeon

Every busy surgeon experiences adverse events during his or her surgical career. When they occur, attention has been directed primarily toward the affected patient. While this is appropriate, and every attempt should be made to minimize patient harm and achieve the best possible outcome expeditiously, the effects of intraoperative adverse events (iAE) upon the surgeon have not received as much discussion as they deserve. Recently, resident and physician wellness, burnout and other similar concerns have received increasing attention. Burnout and depression associated with electronic medical records have been debated widely, and the increasing problem of physician suicide has led to greater sensitivity and resources particularly in graduate medical training institutions. However, the effects of iAEs on the physician have not received as much attention.

In 2017, Han et al.[1] published an interesting article on this topic that provided insights that should be of interest and value to all physicians and especially surgeons. The authors conducted a survey of all surgeons at three major teaching hospitals at the same university. The university was not specified, but the authors reported that it was in Boston. Since all of the authors are from the division of trauma, emergency surgery, and surgical critical care at Massachusetts General Hospital, Harvard Medical School, it seems reasonable to infer that the university studied was of superior quality and reputation. The authors distributed a 29-item questionnaire and received an exceptionally high response rate of 44.8% (126 physicians responding). Some of the findings were somewhat surprising.

The median age of respondents was 49 years, and 77% were male. Over 80% performed more than 150 surgical procedures per year. The survey asked how many iAEs the physicians recalled having experienced within the last year. A surprisingly high 80% reported having experienced an iAE. 32% recalled one, 39% recalled two to five, and 9% recalled six or more iAEs during the preceding twelve months. The responding surgeons admitted to substantial emotional consequences. These included anxiety (60%), guilt (60%), sadness (52%), shame/embarrassment (42%), and anger (29%). Although a few surgeons accepted psychological therapy/counseling, most (42%) reported that colleagues made up their most important support system, not friends or family.

Interestingly and importantly, many iAEs went unreported. More surprisingly, 26% of respondents preferred not to see their personal iAE rates. 38% wanted their iAE rates reported in comparison with the aggregate iAE rates of their colleagues. However, 50% did not report iAEs because of fear of litigation. The other two most common factors for not reporting were lack of a standardized reporting system (49%), and the unavailability of specific definitions of an iAE (48%).

This was essentially the first major study of this important problem, investigating it from the perspective of the surgeon.[1] The fact that 80% of surgeons remembered at least one iAE within the past twelve months is particularly surprising in light of reports that placed the incidence at 1.5-2%, with most of the iAEs being organ lacerations, hemorrhage, and enterotomies.[2] This suggests strongly that the problem is much more widespread than most of us might think, possibly due to factors that prevent physicians from reporting iAEs. Rather than asking the surgeons directly, most previous papers gathered data retrospectively from operative notes that might not have documented iAEs clearly.

It is also clear from this study that iAEs affect surgeons substantially. Surgeons tend to be dedicated perfectionists. Involvement in an iAE takes a great personal and emotional toll. At present, there are exceedingly few peer-support programs that include specific assistance for surgeons or others involved in iAEs.[3,4]

Although the article by Han et al has some limitations including possible response bias, the fact that the study was limited to one university, and the fact that surgical trainees were not included in the study, it should be of considerable interest to all surgeons. First, we should recognize that we are not alone in experiencing an iAE from time to time, and possibly more often than we might have guessed was common. Second, since the published study did not look at various surgical specialties separately, a study of iAEs among surgeons in various fields, and the physicians' response to those iAEs, should be considered. Third, the study clearly reveals that iAEs are underreported.

It is clear that iAEs are underestimated, underreported, and that their impact is underappreciated and undertreated. Surgeons should consider developing a more effective approach to this problem that will be not only not threatening, but moreover constructive.

References

1. Han K, Bohnen JD, Peponis T, et al. The Surgeon as the Second Victim? Results of the Boston Intraoperative Adverse Events Surgeons' Attitude (BISA) Study. *JACS* 2017;224(6):1048–55.
2. Platz J, Hyman N. Tracking intraoperative complications. *JACS* 2012;215:519–23.
3. van Pelt F. Peer support: healthcare professionals supporting each other after adverse medical events. *Qual Saf Health Care* 2008;17:249–52.
4. Hu YY, Fix ML, Hevelone ND, et al. Physicians' needs in coping with emotional stressors: the case for peer support. *Arch Surg* 2012;147:212–17.

Reprinted with modifications by permission of Vendome Group from:
Sataloff RT. Adverse Surgical Events: Effects on the Surgeon. *ENT J*, in press.

53. Geriatric surgery

More than one-third of all inpatient surgical procedures are performed on patients age 65 and over.[1] This is not surprising. In 2015, people ≥65 years constituted 15% of the U.S. population, and this percentage is expected to grow to 24% by 2060.[2] In 2010, nearly 40% of hospital discharges (including short-stay hospitals) involved patients ≥65 years of age.[3] This means that approximately 200 million operations a year are performed on elderly (≥65 years) patients.

We have been trained to understand that pediatric patients are not just 'small adults'. Similarly, geriatric patients are not just 'old adults'. They have special problems and require knowledgeable diagnostic and therapeutic intervention. Emphasizing this issue for example, the American Academy of Otolaryngology-Head and Neck Surgery acknowledged the importance of geriatric otolaryngology by publishing with Thieme a multidisciplinary textbook of geriatric otolaryngology-head and neck surgery in 2015.[4] That text makes it clear that special knowledge of geriatric otolaryngology is important in all subspecialties except pediatric otolaryngology, and such knowledge is especially important in surgical decision making.

On one hand, surgery should not be denied to patients simply because they are 'old'. Moreover, 'old' is hard to define. More and more people are living beyond 100 years, so denying surgery to an 80-year-old and condemning him or her to suffer from a potentially correctable problem for another 15 to 20 years is not right. We need to be concerned about quality of life. On the other hand, surgery that is unlikely to improve quality of life, or that presents a high risk of ending life without a concomitant benefit (such as some surgery for advanced cancer, and some heart surgery), might not be appropriate in this population.

Numerous articles on surgery in the elderly have been published - far too many to reference in this brief chapter. Discussions of this topic appear regularly in publications of the American College of Surgeons, for example. The underlying theme of most of these articles is the need to improve preoperative assessment. Surgical decision-making must focus on more than surgical mortality and morbidity. We must consider maintenance of independence, quality of life, return to at least preoperative functional activity levels, the likely consequences of each person's physiologic reserve, the cognitive effects associated with general anesthesia in the elderly, and the patient's desires regarding quality of life and longevity.

Ideally, with the help of a healthcare team, the surgeon needs to assess and document cognitive function, nutrition, risk of falls, geriatric syndromes, and other special healthcare issues in all elderly patients for whom surgery is contemplated. Such preoperative assessments help not only in surgical decision making, but also in perioperative care of elderly patients.

Elderly patients have increased risk of postoperative morbidity, sometimes after even relatively short general anesthesia. Problems may include long-term cognitive impairment, delirium, deep vein thrombosis, myocardial ischemia, infection, and others. It is essential for the physician, patient, and family to review these risks and make sure everyone agrees that they are justified and weighed against potential benefits. Physician and patient education are required, but much of the necessary knowledge is still being developed.

While there is no specific measure that will guide us in decisions about whether to perform surgery, assessments of frailty can be helpful and enlightening. This topic, as well as other tools for clinical assessment that predict adverse outcomes in geriatric patients, is covered in other literature.[4-10] Interesting studies in geriatric trauma patients have shown the value of frailty assessment. For example, Joseph et al looked at elderly trauma patients (a particularly vulnerable population) and found that a 50-variable frailty index predicted unfavorable discharge disposition in geriatric patients.[11] In a follow-up paper published during the same year, they validated a 15-variable trauma-specific frailty index (TSFI).[12] The TSFI proved to be an effective instrument for predicting discharge disposition in geriatric trauma patients.

Similar studies in many other specialties have not been performed. Other frailty instruments have been used to predict surgical survival and outcomes, although most surgeons (and other physicians) are not using frailty assessment routinely and knowledgably. There are exceptions, such as the University of Pittsburgh Medical Center, where targeted assessments of elderly patients have shown great value.

Nearly all physicians and surgeons care for elderly patients, and the percentage of elderly patients in our practices will continue to increase. It is past time for all surgeons to study specialty-specific implications of advanced age, to apply and study assessment tools that have proven useful in other specialties, and to develop assessments and guidelines to assist us and our trainees in providing optimal care for patients 65 and older.

References

1. Hall MJ, DeFrances CJ, Williams SN, et al. National Hospital Discharge Survey: 2007 summary. National Health Statistics Reports. U.S. Department of Health and Human Services. October 26, 2010. www.cdc.gov/nchs/data/nhsr/nhsr029.pdf. Accessed September 22, 2018.
2. U.S. Census Bureau. 2014 national population projections summary tables. Table 6: Percent distribution of the projected population by sex and selected age groups for the U.S.: 2015 to 2060. www.census.gov/data/tables/2014/demo/popproj/2014-summary-tables.html. Accessed September 22, 2018.
3. Centers for Disease Control and Prevention. Number of discharges from short-stay hospitals, by first-listed diagnosis and age: United States, 2010. www.cdc.gov/nchs/data/nhds/3firstlisted/2010first3_numberage.pdf. Accessed September 22, 2018.
4. Sataloff RT, Johns MM, Kost KM (eds.) Geriatric Otolaryngology. New York, New York:Thieme Medical Publishers and the American Academy of Otolaryngology-Head and Neck Surgery; 2015.
5. Boyd CM, Darer J, Boult C, et al. Clinical practice guidelines and quality of care for older patients with multiple comorbid diseases: Implications for pay for performance. *JAMA* 2005;294(6):716–24.
6. Woods NF, LaCroix AZ, Gray SL, et al. Frailty: Emergence and consequences in women aged 65 and older in the Women's Health Initiative Observational Study. *J Am Geriatr Soc* 2005;53(8):1321–30.
7. Fried LP, Kronmal RA, Newman AB, et al. Risk factors for 5-year mortality in older adults: The Cardiovascular Health Study. *JAMA* 1998;279(8):585–92.
8. Zafonte RD, Hammond FM, Mann NR, et al. Relationship be- tween Glasgow Coma scale and functional outcome. *Am J Phys Med Rehabil* 1996;75(5):364–9.
9. Foreman BP, Caesar RR, Parks J, et al. Usefulness of the abbreviated injury score and the injury severity score in comparison to the Glasgow Coma Scale in predicting outcome after traumatic brain injury. *J Trauma* 2007;62(4):946–50.
10. Shah MK, Al-Adawi S, Burke DT. Age as predictor of functional outcome in anoxic brain injury. *J Appl Res* 2004;4(3):380–4.

11. Joseph B, Pandit V, Rhee P, et al. Predicting hospital discharge disposition in geriatric trauma patients: Is frailty the answer? *J Trauma Acute Care Surgery* 2014;76(1):196–200.
12. Joseph B, Pandit V, Zangbar B, et al. Validating trauma-specific frailty index for geriatric trauma patients: A prospective analysis. *J Am Coll Surg* 2014;219(1):10–17.

Reprinted with modifications by permission of Vendome Group from:
Sataloff RT. Geriatric surgery in otolaryngology. *ENT J* 2018;97(3):50–2.

54. Telemedicine

John S. Rubin, M.D., F.A.C.S., F.R.C.S.
Consultant Otolaryngologist, Royal National Throat Nose and Ear Hospital; Honorary Consultant Otolaryngologist, National Hospital for Neurology and Neurosurgery, University College London Hospitals NHS Trust; Honorary Visiting Professor, School of Health Sciences, City University of London, Honorary Senior Lecturer, Department of Surgery, University College London

Robert T. Sataloff, M.D., D.M.A., F.A.C.S.
Professor and Chairman, Department of Otolaryngology–Head and Neck Surgery; Senior Associate Dean for Clinical Academic Specialties, Drexel University College of Medicine

The concept of remote medicine has generated increasing interest in recent years. Telemedicine is the provision of healthcare, consultation, and/or information using electronic communications technology.

Broad categories of telemedicine include (1) 'store and forward', (2) remote monitoring, and (3) real-time interactive services. It is useful for otolaryngologists to understand all three options.

Store and forward involves acquisition and review of medical data. This might include materials such as medical images or biosignals. It allows for the transmission of medical data off site, thereby permitting review at the convenience of the expert. There is no requirement for the two parties (patient and provider) to be present synchronously. For example, radiologists use this approach routinely. Images are acquired at point A, sent to point B, reported on by the radiologist at point B, and the results are returned to the initiating provider of services at point A or elsewhere, or simply stored for later interpretation or use. Histopathology is another service that uses this approach. There are potential applications for numerous other noninvasive bioimage acquisitions and interpretations.

Remote monitoring implies off-site monitoring of medical problems. It is particularly apt for chronic disease review that does not require face-to-face assessment. It has been used to monitor conditions such as diabetes, emphysema and chronic obstructive pulmonary disease, asthma, and congestive heart failure. A few reports have suggested that under carefully controlled circumstances, this type of remote monitoring has health outcomes comparable to face-to-face monitoring.[1-5]

Real-time interactive services can theoretically exist between patient and provider via phone, online, and in 'kiosks'. One suggested approach is a 'health spot', perhaps located in a pharmacy or large department store, where a patient could enter and interact remotely with a physician. This examination booth or kiosk would be supplied with a variety of medical devices that could be monitored remotely. The physician could also be available on a real-time basis via a video-televised link for direct face-to-face history taking and discussion.

American Well Online Care is an online care delivery service that offers such a service via chat, voice, and video. Physicians can sign up for the service and thereby provide the patient and/or another physician with immediate consultation.[6] American Well has launched a 'direct-to-consumer' service with live video consultations available in 44 U.S. states and the District of Columbia.[7]

Early systematic reviews[4,5] found the strongest evidence for the efficacy of telemedicine in clinical outcomes from home-based care and monitoring applications in the areas of chronic disease management, hypertension, and AIDS (although Hersh et al noted that evidence of value of home glucose monitoring in diabetes mellitus was conflicting).[4] They also found what they described as 'reasonable evidence' that telemedicine is comparable to face-to-face care in emergency medicine and is beneficial in surgical and neonatal intensive care units, as well as patient transfer in neurosurgery.

Hersh et al cautioned that there is only a small amount of evidence that interventions provided by telemedicine result in clinical outcomes comparable to or better than face-to-face care and recommended larger randomized, controlled trials.[4]

It has been argued that telemedicine is cost-effective and might be associated with greater patient satisfaction. In 2012, the Ontario Telemedicine Network[2] summarized self-reported data from 813 enrolled patients with congestive heart disease and chronic obstructive pulmonary disease, noting a 64 to 66% decrease in hospital admissions, a 72 to 74% reduction in emergency department visits, a 16 to 33% decrease in primary care physician visits, and a 95 to 97% decrease in walk-in clinic visits.[2]

Others are less convinced. De Jongh et al performed a Cochrane review of mobile phone messaging for facilitating self-management of long-term illnesses.[8] They concluded that there were some, albeit limited, indications that mobile phone messaging interventions may provide benefit in supporting the self-management of long-term illnesses. However, they noted significant information gaps regarding the long-term effects, acceptability, costs, and risks of such interventions.

Baron et al, looking at mobile management technologies on glycosylated hemoglobin of patients with diabetes, summarized in their abstract that the evidence on the effectiveness of *mhealth* (mobile health technologies) interventions for diabetes 'was inconsistent for both types of diabetes and remains weak' in the studies that they reviewed.[9]

Smith et al performed a cost-benefit analysis for a telepediatric service in Queensland.[10] They demonstrated the service to be financially viable over a 5-year program but found start-up costs to be considerable and to represent 40% of the entire 5-year costs. Stensland et al, in contrast, found a cost excess in a telemedical outpatient program in Minnesota.[11] This was primarily due to cost of personnel and an increase in the volume of specialty care and in the use of specialty services by the patients.

Henderson et al, in the recent Whole Systems Demonstrator program, found total costs associated with the telehealth intervention side to be higher than those associated with traditional face-to-face contact.[12] Davalos et al pointed out that economic evaluations of telemedicine remain rare, and few of those conducted have accounted for the wide range of economic costs and benefits.[13]

Benefits that have been suggested from telemedicine include an increase in productivity, increase in speed of processes and referrals, and increased ease in interaction among patients, medical, and paramedical personnel. It has also been argued that such services allow for lower costs of health care. Arguments made by service providers include the benefits for remote environs and elimination of the need to travel long distances.

As one example, Massachusetts General Hospital and Brigham and Women's Hospital offer a 'Partner Telestroke Center'. This center offers collaboration via brain imaging review, remote examination via video conferencing, and a Web portal for synchronized store-and-forward requirements.[14]

By way of clinical examples, a 2012 Guest Editorial for *Ear, Nose & Throat Journal* outlined ENT-related usages of telemedicine.[15] Some examples included: Louisiana in the aftermath of Hurricane Katrina, where a telemedicine service was developed for neurotology patients,[16] and Anchorage, Alaska, where a remote video-otoscopy service had been devised for post-tympanotomy tube insertion patients.[17] There are several potential benefits of telemedicine for patients with voice disorders and their providers, including remote readings of strobovideolaryngoscopic and high-speed imaging, as well as provision of voice therapy.[18]

Telemedicine has several issues that still must be addressed if it is to become a pillar of medical care. Initial issues included difficulty in use, expense, limited reach, and slowness of service. Many of these issues have been resolved as technology has improved. Concerns regarding patient confidentiality, security, and regulatory challenges remain, however. Reimbursement issues also are still problematic in many areas, placing the investment burden on the hospital healthcare system or physician. Furthermore, cultural barriers are not easy to overcome as patients and doctors need to adapt to telemedicine paradigms for most effective use of the new techniques.

There also are legal issues that remain a substantial impediment, especially in the United States, where medical licensure is on a state-by-state basis. Problematic examples can be envisioned readily. For example, if a physician is performing a remote examination on a patient who is physically in the state of California while the physician is working in and only licensed to practice medicine in the state of New York, is the physician liable for practicing medicine in California without a license? At present, the answer is yes. Location of practice is defined as the location of the patient, not the physician.

Clarification also is required for analysis of biosignals, such as radiologic examinations that are stored in one state but reviewed in another. Similar queries could be posited for physicians practicing remotely between countries.

As of the time of writing this chapter, the underlying suppositions that telemedicine is cost-effective and that it improves well-being are still unproven. The Whole System Demonstrator Programme was launched by Great Britain's Department of Health in May 2008. It is the largest randomized, controlled trial of telehealth and telecare in the United Kingdom, involving (according to the Department of Health in its 'Early Headline Findings')[19] 6,191 patients and 238 general practices across three sites: Newham, Kent, and Cornwall. In total, 3,030 people with one of three conditions (diabetes, heart failure, or chronic obstructive pulmonary disease) were included in the telehealth trial. For the telecare element of the trial, people were selected using the Fair Access to Care Services criteria.[19]

The results are still being analyzed. The UK Department of Health states: 'If used correctly, telehealth can deliver a 15% reduction in A&E [accident and emergency department] visits, a 20% reduction in emergency admissions, a 14% reduction in elective admissions, a 14% reduction in bed days, and an 8% reduction in tariff costs. More strikingly…a 45% reduction in mortality rates'.[19]

In 2012, Steventon et al described 179 general practices and 3,230 people with diabetes, chronic obstructive pulmonary disease, or heart failure recruited from practices between May 2008 and November 2009 and concluded that telehealth is associated with lower mortality and emergency admission rates.[20] The reasons for the short-term increases in admissions for the control group are not clear, but the trial recruitment processes could have had an effect. However, as Gornall stated, 'Whether telehealth can help to reduce NHS costs, chiefly by reducing admissions and freeing up beds for closure, remains a complex question'.[21]

The BBC website, on March 21, 2013, ran the headline, 'NHS remote monitoring 'costs more'.'[22] In this article, they stated, 'The cost per quality-adjusted life year-a combined measure of quantity and quality of life of telehealth-was £92,000 when added to usual care. This is way above the threshold of £30,000 that the National Institute for Health and Clinical Excellence has set. A best-case scenario considering that the price of equipment was likely to fall over time and that services were not running at full capacity during the trial, saw the probability that the service was cost-effective rise from 11% to 61%'.

In 2016, Gunter et al published a systematic review of the current use of telemedicine for post-discharge surgical care.[23] Their review provided 72 references, including seven articles that studied clinical outcomes associated with telemedicine. All reported either no difference in the numbers of complications in the telemedicine group versus the group receiving usual care, or slightly higher complication rates in the telemedicine group, although they could not relate those complications causally to the use of telemedicine. The greatest financial savings noted in their review accrued to the patients, particularly savings related to travel time and costs, although savings to healthcare systems were found, as well.

The role of telemedicine is increasing. Newer technologies such as mobile phone messaging applications, short message service, and multimedia message service have become readily available. Such technologies lend themselves to telemedical approaches. However, the future standing of telemedicine in medicine in general and in otolaryngology specifically remains unclear.

References

1. Department of Health. Whole system demonstrator programme: Headline findings. December 2011. https://www.gov.uk/government/publications/whole-system-demonstrator-programme-headline-findings-december-2011. Accessed June 11, 2018.
2. OTN Telemedicine's Leader. 2013. http://www.otn.ca
3. Rendina MC, Downs SM, Carasco N, et al. Effect of telemedicine on health outcomes in 87 infants requiring neonatal intensive care. *Telemed J* 1998;4(4):345–51.
4. Hersh WR, Helfand M, Wallace J, et al. Clinical outcomes resulting from telemedicine interventions: A systematic review. *BMC Med Inform Decis Mak* 2001;1:5.
5. Hailey D, Roine R, Ohinmaa A. Systematic review of evidence for the benefits of telemedicine. *J Telemed Telecare* 2002;8(Suppl 1):1–30.
6. American Well Online Care. https://www.Americanwell.com. Accessed June 11, 2018.
7. Terry K. American Well: The doctor will see you online. Information Week. October 8, 2013. www.informationweek.com/mobile/american-well-the-doctor-will-see-you-online/d/d-id/1111870. Accessed June 8, 2018.
8. de Jongh T, Gurol-Urganci I, Vodopivec-Jamsek V, et al. Mobile phone messaging for facilitating self-management of long-term illnesses. *Cochrane Database Syst Rev* 2012;12:CD007459.
9. Baron J, McBain H, Newman S. The impact of mobile monitoring technologies on glycosylated hemoglobin in diabetes: A systematic review. *J Diabetes Sci Technol* 2012;6(5):1185–96.
10. Smith AC, Scuffham P, Wootton R. The costs and potential savings of a novel telepaediatric service in Queensland. *BMC Health Serv Res* 2007;7:35.
11. Stensland J, Speedie SM, Ideker M, et al. The relative cost of outpatient telemedicine services. *Telemed J* 1999;5(3):245–56.
12. Henderson C, Knapp M, Fernández JL, et al. Cost effectiveness of telehealth for patients with long term conditions (Whole Systems Demonstrator telehealth questionnaire study): Nested economic evaluation in a pragmatic, cluster randomised controlled trial. *BMJ* 2013; 346:f1035.
13. Dávalos ME, French MT, Burdick AE, Simmons SC. Economic evaluation of telemedicine: Review of the literature and research guidelines for benefit-cost analysis. *Telemed J E Health* 2009;15(10):933–48.

14. Massachusetts General Hospital Stroke Service. 2013. https://telestroke.massgeneral.org/default.asp. Accessed June 11, 2018.
15. Garritano FG, Goldenberg D. Telemedicine in otolaryngology-head and neck surgery. *Ear Nose Throat J* 2012;91(6):226–9.
16. Arriaga MA, Nuss D, Scrantz K, et al. Telemedicine- assisted neurotology in post-Katrina Southeast Louisiana. *Otol Neurotol* 2010;31(3):524–7.
17. Kokesh J, Ferguson AS, Patricoski C, et al. Digital images for postsurgical follow-up of tympanostomy tubes in remote Alaska. *Otolaryngol Head Neck Surg* 2008;139(1):87–93.
18. Rubin J, Sataloff RT, Korovin G. Telemedicine. In: *Diagnosis and Treatment of Voice Disorders*, 4th edition. San Diego, California: Plural Publishing, Inc.; 2014:781–4.
19. Department of Health. Whole System Demonstrator Programme: Headline findings. December 2011. https://www.gov.uk/government/publications/whole-system-demonstrator-programme-headline-findings-december-2011. Accessed June 11, 2018.
20. Steventon A, Bardsley M, Billings J, et al. Effect of telehealth on use of secondary care and mortality: Findings from the Whole System Demonstrator cluster randomised trial. *BMJ* 2012;344:e3874.
21. Gornall J. Does telemedicine deserve the green light? *BMJ* 2012;345:e4622.
22. No authors listed. NHS remote monitoring 'costs more.' BBC News. March 21, 2013. www.bbc.co.uk/news/health-21874978. Accessed July 12, 2018.
23. Gunter RL, Chouinard S, Fernandes-Taylor S, et al. Current use of telemedicine for post-discharge surgical care: A systematic review. *J Am Coll Surg* 2016;225(5):915–27.

Reprinted with modifications by permission of Plural Publishing, Inc. from:
    Rubin, J., Sataloff, R.T. and Korovin, G. *Diagnosis and Treatment of Voice Disorders*, 4th Edition. San Diego, California: Plural Publishing, Inc. 2014; pp. 981–984.

55. The aging physician and surgeon

Robert T. Sataloff, M.D., D.M.A., F.A.C.S.
Mary Hawkshaw, RN, BSN, CORLN
Joshua Kutinsky, J.D., Psy.D.
Edward A. Maitz, Ph.D.

Introduction

As the percentage of elderly people in our population increases, so does the percentage of elderly physicians. Older doctors, some practicing part-time or in a restricted capacity, might be part of the solution to the expected shortage of health care providers. However, it is essential to ensure that practicing physicians remain competent. The need for assessing functional competence has been recognized and studied, especially among surgeons. However, the lack of accepted methods for evaluation and criteria for determining the functional correlates of physician competence has created practical and legal difficulties. These challenges also are particularly apparent among surgeons.

Hospitals are obligated to assure the competence and qualifications of their medical staffs. Most rely on department chairs to review applications for surgical privileges (initial applications and frequent reapplications). Credentials committees generally accept the endorsement of department chairs. However, those of us who are department chairs frequently face daunting challenges in evaluating and attesting to the competence of aging surgeons.

In most institutions, there are no objective measures used routinely to assess manual or cognitive functions. Hence, judgments by department chairs are based on personal observation and impressions; opinions expressed by trainees, nurses, and others who are in the operating room; and in some cases, by outcome data. Denying privileges on the basis of a clinical impression of decreasing competence is difficult, especially when the aging surgeon in question was a mentor to the current department chair.

In addition, the aging surgeon may not recognize a change in function; and denial of privileges without objective information can lead not only to acrimony, but also to lawsuits for age and employment discrimination. Unfortunately, the documentation available to us usually is an increased prevalence of bad outcomes. It seems self-evident that if we wait to take action until after a previously excellent surgeon has been sued repeatedly for bad outcomes, then we have waited too long and have failed to protect the patients, hospital, and the aging surgeon.

This article from which this chapter is derived was started because of the senior author's (RTS) belief that it should be possible to promulgate an efficient, valid, reliable assessment protocol that could be used widely, would provide objective data on relevant human performance, and that would generate data that correlated with patient outcomes and delivery of safe medical care. It also seemed curious to the author that this problem had not been addressed more fully previously. As the following literature review demonstrates, it has been studied, at least to a degree. However, none of the proposals or methodologies has been adopted widely, and most physicians (surgeons and others) are not familiar with the literature.

While this article deals primarily with surgeons because they have been studied most widely, and with pilots for whom assessment using cognitive and manual function is more advanced than it is for surgeons, the principles apply to physicians in all specialties. This chapter provides a fairly comprehensive review of existing literature, as well as a proposal for development of a routine assessment protocol for physicians as we age.

Materials and methods

MEDLINE and PubMed databases were searched using articles from 1960 to the present. Search terms included *aging, aging physician, geriatric physician*, and *aging surgeon*. A total of 14,562 articles were identified, and abstracts of potentially relevant articles were reviewed. Many anecdotal opinion articles were excluded, although a few particularly insightful such commentaries were referenced. Selected additional important references cited in the selected articles also were reviewed, as were articles on aging pilots that appear to be relevant to the problems of aging physicians.

In addition, common neuropsychological tests were reviewed, and a protocol was suggested for longitudinal screening of cognitive function in physicians. Additional research and correlation of cognitive data with physician performance is recommended to determine if/how cognitive test results can be used in evaluating aging physicians and predicting clinically relevant changes in function.

Review of the literature

In a 1983 commentary in *JAMA*, Bunkin offered a personal account of his feelings of unpreparedness when he had reached age 60 and had not given any previous consideration to retirement.[1] He discussed the need for surgeons to be alert for subtle and insidious signs of degradation in their surgical performance. At approximately age 67, Bunkin reviewed his operative times and noted that each operation had taken approximately 20 minutes longer than similar procedures had required during the previous year. He stated that 'technical know-how was intact, but the movements in sequence were each several seconds longer'. He described omitting a step in an operative procedure that he had performed more than 3,000 times over a span of 36 years. Dr. Bunkin stated that he found these changes in his performance as a surgeon 'unexpectedly scary', and they initiated his consideration of retirement. He added, 'If you are in good health, the prognosis for a fulfilling retirement is very good'.

Greenfield and Proctor conducted a survey to examine the attitudes and practices surrounding retirement in a group of senior surgeons in 1993.[2] Their survey was mailed to 882 members of the American Surgical Association, and 659 (75%) returned their responses. The survey contained questions related to age which was broken down into >40, >50, >60, and >70 years; plans for retirement; work load or operative activity; and withdrawal from privileges (age, disability, and peer review).

Forty percent of all responders reported no retirement plans. In the age group 40 to 50 there were 46 responders, and only 3 reported having a plan for retirement. In the 60 to 70 age group there were 211 responders; 49 reported having a plan for retirement, and 75 reported no plan for retirement. The limitations of this study are age and gender. Most of the respondents were of senior age and male. The survey results showed some evidence of retirement planning with advancing age, but not among all surgeons.

The surgeon responders also were asked to describe their level of surgical activity, and the majority reported a decline in their workload between ages 60 and 70. However, 40% reported a customary workload past 60 years of age. Seventy-two percent of the responders thought that decisions regarding when privileges to operate are withdrawn should be based on peer review or the onset of a disability. The authors suggested that more positive attitudes towards retirement were needed. They advocated the development of methods for performance evaluation that would reflect the surgeon's response to his or her personal aging. They also pointed out that 'both personal and institutional problems can arise when surgeons continue to practice despite limitation of aging'.

In 1993, as president of the International Society for Cardiovascular Surgery, Lazar Greenfield delivered his presidential address titled 'Farewell to Surgery'.[3] The focus of his discussion was the performance of aging surgeons and the impact of the end of mandatory retirement. He noted that there was little known about behaviors of aging surgeons but that there had been a great deal of interest in older workers in general with regard to productivity and job safety. He pointed out that the science of applied ergonomics defines an 'older worker' as anyone over the age of 40 and stated that studies have shown that age 40 is the time of onset of performance slowing, decrease in ability to learn new skills, decline in motivation and creativity, and one's ability to cope with stress and change.[4,5]

Greenfield provided an excellent review of the physiology of aging highlighting its complexity and its effect on multiple organs and systems in both males and females. He discussed the decline in vision, hearing, mobility, and dexterity that occurs in everyone over time; and he pointed out that physical strength and joint flexibility diminish, as well as overall elasticity of leg and arm movements. He commented that studies have shown reduced motion of the lumbar spine and slowing of nerve conduction in the elderly. He cited one report that showed an age-related reduction in the ability to diffuse lactate during strenuous exercise beginning as early as age 30, thus contributing to overall decreased endurance.[6]

Dr. Greenfield discussed The Age Discrimination in Employment Act of 1967[7] that prohibits mandatory retirement based on age. He pointed out that there were nevertheless a few professional organizations that still mandated retirement at a specific age including the Federal Aviation Administration (FAA) (age 65) and the Federal Bureau of Investigation (FBI) (age 57). U.S. Congress has approved mandatory retirement ages for several other professions that involve public safety including air traffic controllers (age 56), light house operators (age 55), and national park rangers (age 57).[8]

Greenfield discussed the FAA's previous mandatory retirement at age 60 for commercial pilots and the concept of calculated risk.[9] The Fair Treatment for Experienced Pilots Act was signed into law in 2007 raising the mandatory retirement age for pilots to 65.[10,11]

A pilot's performance and outcome can affect a larger number of people, whereas a surgeon's ability to perform poses potential risk to one person (at a time). Moreover, Greenfield recognized that historically surgeons and all physicians have focused on the knowledge and competency that are measured in order to begin the practice of medicine, highlighting that little attention has been paid to when it is time to stop practicing.

Greenfield discussed the federal highway safety standard that requires licensed drivers to undergo reexamination at least every 4 years. This examination includes test of visual acuity and knowledge. He commented on the sensitive issue of age discrimination in the United States and the need to avoid bias against the elderly even when it comes to operating a motor vehicle, pointing out that 'the public can legitimately ask why is it that the older individual must take examinations to be able to drive but not to be an operating surgeon'. He pointed out that many public policies use age-based criteria such as eligibility for Medicare and Social Security, tax benefits, and the federal laws that do not allow an individual to get a driver's license before age 16 or purchase alcoholic beverages before age 21.

Greenfield discussed cognitive function in older physicians and the development of a computerized neuropsychological screening battery Assessment of Cognitive Function developed by Powell.[12] Greenfield suggested that cognitive and functional testing should be performed under controlled situations so that objective data can be used in establishing performance criteria. He stated that more research was needed and longitudinal rather than cross-sectional studies should be used to gain better data regarding aging surgeons and performance.

Trunkey and Botney's review article published in 2001 compared how surgeons assess age-related competence and how commercial aviation assesses pilots' competency.[13] The authors cited a publication by James B. Stewart in which he stated, 'Five out of every 100 doctors are so incompetent, drunk, senile, or otherwise impaired that they should not be practicing medicine without some form of restriction', and that the 'quality-improvement process is seriously flawed and has not been effective in weeding out incompetent physicians'.[14] The authors pointed out that Stewart's opinions were expressed in a book and were not the conclusions of a peer-reviewed study.

The *American Heritage Dictionary* defines competency as 'the quality or condition of being legally qualified, eligible or admissible'.[15] The authors point out that skills, ability, and performance are not that same as competence and lack legal implication. They state that, historically, the medical profession has used volume performance and outcomes as a measure of competency; however, 'neither have the same meaning nor have they withstood scientific scrutiny'.

Trunkey and Botney pointed out that determining a surgeon's competence as he or she ages is complex and multifactorial. They discussed factors including reaction time, decision-making time, cognitive decline, decline in psychomotor skills, dysfunctional or antisocial behavior, substance abuse, and the failure to keep learning. The authors reviewed a book by Douglas H. Powell titled *Profiles in Cognitive Aging* that outlined multiple changes in cognitive function, physiology, and psychometrics that occur with aging.[12]

Powell developed a series of assessments called the MicroCog test to measure and document these changes. The tests were not designed to evaluate expert knowledge but rather to examine attention, reaction time, numerical recall, verbal memory, visuospatial facility, reasoning, and mental calculation. Powell reported MicroCog test results of 1002 physicians and 581 normal subjects which showed progressive, age-related decline in both groups.

Trunkey and Botney reported that the tests of reactivity, simple reaction time, and choice reaction time were useful in measuring decline in surgeon performance. They suggested that 'in general, a simple reaction time does not consistently correlate with performance' and that 'choice reaction time may discriminate experts from novices but does not do so consistently'.

Trunkey and Botney also discussed the Federal Bureau of Investigation's (FBI) test for assessing reaction time and performance, which utilizes a simulator that presents threat situations to evaluate an agent's accuracy and reaction time.[16] The authors pointed out that rapid decisions and action are required of trauma surgeons, much like FBI agents in the field, but in medicine, there was no simulator to test decision making ability of surgeons. Today, simulators with such capabilities exist; but they have not been studied sufficiently to determine their ability to validly detect age related decrement in surgical ability. Hence, they are not in wide use or relied upon for assessment of surgeons.

The authors also compared surgery and aviation. Newly trained surgeons have their competency assessed through board certification in their specialty following successful completion of a residency program. Board certification is regarded as a fairly good assessment of a surgeon's competence. The authors pointed out that many surgeons are required to recertify every 10 years. Part of recertification includes an affidavit from the chief surgeon at his/her institution stating that the applicant for recertification has not been treated for drug/substance abuse; not had his or her license revoked or restricted; not been censored by the American College of Surgeons, their hospital or state society; and has not been convicted of a felony. The statement does not include an endorsement of surgical competency; and if it did, making negative judgment would be challenging medically and legally for the chief surgeon and hospital because of the absence of standard objective instruments to evaluate an aging surgeon's performance and consensus in how the assessment results should be used.

Pilots undergo medical certification every 6 months are subject to random blood and urinalysis screening for substance abuse. The pilots' medical evaluation is extensive, and there are several conditions that can disqualify a pilot from flying including but not limited to: insulin dependent diabetes, angina, coronary artery disease, myocardial infarction, heart valve replacement, heart transplant, and cardiac pacemaker placement. Pilots undergo simulator testing at least annually, and commercial airline pilots are subjected to 'unannounced checkouts' by the FAA. Retirement at age 60 was mandated by the FAA[9] until 2007 when the age was raised to 65.[11]

The authors discussed the need to address impaired competence late in a surgeon's career. They proposed medical evaluation and certification beginning at age 50, then every 2 years to age 60, then annually after age 60. They suggested employing MicroCog testing, random breathalyzer and urine screening, and increasing the frequency of recertification.

In 2006, Waljee et al examined surgeon age and operative mortality in the United States.[17] Using the national Medicare files, they reviewed the operative mortality in more than 400,000 patients who had undergone one of 8 surgical procedures between 1998 and 1999. Operative mortality was defined as in the hospital or within 30 days of surgery. They categorized surgeon age into 4 groups: ≤40 years, 41 to 50 years, 51 to 60 years, and >60 years of age. Mortality rates of 8 different surgical procedures were examined including: pancreatectomy, coronary artery bypass grafting, carotid endarterectomy, esophagectomy, cystectomy, lung resection, aortic valve replacement, and aortic aneurysm repair.

In the analysis of surgeon age and operative mortality, the authors reported that Odds Ratio (OR) and Confidence Interval (CI) adjustments were made for each surgery performed. They found that surgeons over 60 years of age who had low procedure volumes had higher mortality rates compared with younger surgeons. Additionally, they found that the age of a surgeon was not an indicator of operative risk.

Hummer pointed out that there is no age-based definition of physical competence that exists in the United States.[18] He stated that U.S. case law exists primarily due to the Age Discrimination in Employment Act (ADEA) of 1967, which protects individuals over 40 years of age from employment discrimination based on age.[7] He stated that according to the Federation of State Medical Boards (FSMB) in the United States, advanced age is not considered a disqualification for an unrestricted medical license in any state. However, he pointed out that some states do have a minimum age requirement for obtaining licensure.

Dr. Hummer discussed the difficulty in the objective analysis of a surgeon's skill. He pointed out that objective tools such as computer-generated virtual reality and live animal surgery that examine manual dexterity, surgical decision making, and procedure-specific technical skills were in early stages of development in 2007. In assessing surgical competence and when it ends, Hummer suggested that physicians should 'police our own' and determine the criteria rather than being subject to a regulatory entity outside of medicine making such determinations.

Dr. Hummer added that from a surgeon's perspective, retiring from the practice of surgery can be considered a negative life transition due to the loss of the role of being a surgeon.

Blasier reviewed the effects of aging on the physical and cognitive performance of surgeons.[19] He stated, 'For a while, advance in age is accompanied by increasing wisdom: however, eventually even mentation declines'. He considered the question of whether or not older surgeons make 'difficult surgery more difficult or risky surgery riskier?' Dr. Blasier discussed the number of years between a surgeon's completion of medical training and residency and the chronologic age of the practicing surgeon. Considering that most surgeons complete residency and enter practice in their early 30s, Blasier suggested that 'remoteness of any surgeon's initial education can be estimated as his/her age minus 31 years'. Moreover, he pointed out that the content of medical education and training has changed over time.

As an example, Blasier stated that in the practice of orthopedic surgery nearly 'every treatment technique taught 25 years ago has been abandoned and replaced'. Knee and hip replacement procedures have changed dramatically in recent years. Blasier stated that any surgeon 66 years or older would not have received any training in these procedures during his/her residency and that surgeons 40 years of age and older would not have been trained in residency in the current techniques of joint replacement. He pointed out further that all surgical subspecialties undergo changes in treatment and techniques that require changes in the surgeon's skill set. Blasier noted that a few studies have examined the relationship between the surgeon's age and the time when medical training and residency was completed.[20-23]

Research over the past few decades has documented that aging causes deterioration in physical and cognitive skill,[12,24-29] and surgeons need to be aware of signs in declining performance. Blasier stressed that, in general, surgeons have been reluctant to plan for retirement; and he cited Rovit's reasons that surgeons forestall consideration of retirement including fear of death, lack of self-esteem, and resistance to change.[30]

Blasier also discussed that in the United States there is no federally mandated retirement age for surgeons. In the United Kingdom, surgeons in the public health service were mandated to stop performing surgery at age 65 and retire from practice at age 70, until 2011 when the United Kingdom phased out mandatory retirement at age 65 for all professions.[31-33]

In 2008, researchers from the University of Michigan reported results of their study on neuropsychological test performance in surgeons.[34] They compared the performance of 4th-year medical students at the University of Michigan who had matched into their surgical residency program (n = 21) with a group of practicing surgeons (n = 308) between the ages of 45 to 75 years who attended the American College of Surgeons Clinical Congress between the years 2001 and 2004.

The surgeon group was divided further into 2 groups: ages 45 to 60 (n = 139) and ages 61 to 75 (n = 169). They used the Cambridge Neuropsychological Test Automated Battery (CANTAB) to examine psychomotor and visual spatial abilities in the participants.[35,36] They found a decline in performance with aging. The medical student group performed better that the surgeon group aged 45 to 60, and the surgeon group aged 45 to 60 performed better than the surgeon group age 61 to 75. They reported that all three groups performed better than their normative control groups. They concluded that psychomotor and visual-spatial abilities do not improve over time with surgical training and that they are present before one enters medical practice.

Limitations of the University of Michigan study included the inability to assess the impact of surgical experience on procedural learning ability and the limited size of the medical student group. The authors pointed out that there has been increased interest in the impact of aging on procedural learning abilities, and they recommend further longitudinal studies. We also note another shortcoming: There is no evidence in this study to determine the relationship between the psychomotor and visual-spatial skills studied and surgical outcomes.

Bieliauskas et al examined age, cognition, and retirement in a group of senior surgeons.[37] They titled their study using the acronym CCRASS (cognitive changes and retirement among senior surgeons). Their study was designed to identify parameters of cognitive aging in senior surgeons and the relationship to a surgeon's decision to retire.

The CCRASS study included a computerized battery of cognitive tasks that focused on visual learning, sustained attention, and reaction time. Participants also were asked to complete a self- report survey, defining their surgical practice and plans for retirement. The study participants were surgeons 45 years of age and older who attended the annual meeting of the American College of Surgeons from 2001 to 2006.

A total of 359 surgeon volunteers (330 males, 29 females) were tested between 2001 and 2005, and 94 participants were retested in 2005 and 2006. 294 participants completed the survey. The mean age of participants was 61.4 years of age, and 62 surgeons reported that they had already retired.

The author's computerized cognitive testing of the participants utilized 3 subtests from the CANTAB battery of tests, including PAL (paired associates learning), RTI (reaction time), and RVIP (rapid visual information processing).

The CCRASS study showed an age-related decline in all cognitive tasks measured. The authors reported a significant relationship between a surgeon's subjective awareness of cognitive changes and retirement status, but no significant relationship between subjective and objective measurements of cognition. The authors concluded that their study 'supports the need for development of measures of functional aging that can be used over time to assist with decisions about retirement that are in the best interest of surgeons and the patients that they serve.'

In a report published in 2010, Drag et al discussed the results from the CCRASS study and their examination of objective cognitive function in senior surgeons in relation to age and retirement status.[38] The authors administered a computerized cognitive testing battery to a group of surgeons (n = 294), both practicing and retired. Based on age, the participants were divided into two groups: age <60 (n = 126) and age 60 and above (n = 168). Cognitive testing measured 3 tasks including attention, reaction time, and visual learning and memory. The results were compared between the two groups. The authors found that the majority (61%) of practicing surgeons age 60 and older performed within the same range as the surgeons less than 60 years of age on all three tasks measured. Seven of the 108 surgeons over age 60 performed significantly below the younger group of surgeons on more than one task. The authors also found that 'age was negatively correlated with cognitive performance' and that the results showed variability in cognitive performance in the group of older surgeons. The authors concluded that 'age alone cannot predict cognitive competence'.

An article by pediatric neurosurgeon and past president of the AMA, Peter Carmel, MD, discussed aging physicians and retirement.[39] Carmel pointed out that traditionally, physicians 'keep on working as long as we can' for multiple reasons including personal satisfaction, emotional stimulation, and economic or financial need. He stated that retirement for physicians has generally meant reducing office hours and/or reducing the amount or types of surgeries performed.

At age 75, Dr. Carmel stated that he would find slowing down difficult in his surgical practice. He pointed out that the high costs of medical malpractice premiums and the cost of licensing are factors influencing surgeons' need to continue working full-time. Internists and general practitioners often continue working full-time since 'there is simply no one to take over their patient load'.

Carmel pointed out that Americans are living longer than previous generations, and this has resulted in a larger population of senior citizens. He stated, 'This country is facing a shortage of doctors to meet the needs of our growing and aging population'. He stated further that senior physicians will 'play a crucial role in filling this gap' and that the AMA will have an active role in 'accessing, relicensing, and credentialing senior physicians in the future'.

An article in the *New York Times* by Laurie Tarkan addressed concerns regarding physician performance with advancing age.[40] She stated that approximately 20% of physicians were over 65 years of age in 2008 according to AMA data, and that baby boomers are more likely to delay retirement at age 65 due to financial pressures and the current state of our nation's economy, the fact that Social Security benefits may be in jeopardy, and the need for seniors to purchase secondary personal health insurance in addition to Medicare. She pointed out that there is no standard measurement of competency and neurocognitive abilities in surgeons and that physicians and colleagues often do not recognize problems or changes in the aging physician's performance until something bad happens, such as the death of a patient. She advocated medical and cognitive evaluation on a regular basis similar to the FAA's requirements for pilots, pointing out that renewing medical licensure to practice requires completion and documentation of CMEs only. She advocated the need for more research to define an assessment process.

In 2013, the American College of Surgeons Board of Governors Committee on Physician Competency and Health published a set of guidelines, Being Well and Staying Competent: Challenges for the Surgeon, that is available to members of the American College of Surgeons at **www.efacs.org**.

The aging surgeon and determining when it is time to retire from practice was addressed by Garrett and Kaups in a 2014 *Bulletin of the American College of Surgeons*.[41] Their article is an excerpt from the ACS guidelines published in 2013 as stated above. The authors discuss the impact of aging on cognition and performance of surgeons and remind us that there is no mandated retirement age for surgeons, unlike pilots and FBI agents. They discussed the role of objective assessment of surgical skills and judgment, the reliability of self-evaluation of skills and judgment, a surgeon's opinion on when to retire, and the small number of surgeons who plan for retirement.

Garrett and Kaups point out that surgeons, as a profession, need to assure the public of the delivery of safe care. The authors recommend psychomotor assessment and periodic medical evaluation of practicing surgeons between the ages of 62 and 75 years. They report that Stanford University Medical Center enacted a policy recently that requires physicians on staff age 75 and older to 'have a physical examination, cognitive screening, and peer assessment of…clinical performance every 2 years'; and that 'if the findings point to potential concern for patient safety, the service chief and credentials committee will, on a confidential basis, consider the results and recommend further evaluation as necessary'.[42] Additionally, Garrett and Kaups recommended that surgeons plan for the transition from active surgical practice both professionally and financially.

Sun reported in 2014 that, in addition to Stanford's enactment of age related (<75 years) screening of physical health and cognition, a few other institutions across the United States have implemented similar programs, including Driscoll Children's Hospital in Corpus Christi, Texas, and University of Virginia Health System.[43] Sun commented that according to national health care consultant Jonathan Burroughs, 'Only 5% of more than 900 U.S. hospitals with which he has consulted have any active policy for screening older providers'.

Sun pointed out that aging physicians and retirement age have been addressed outside the United States, as well. He stated that the mandatory retirement age for the physicians in Pakistan is 70 years, and in India retirement is mandated at age 65. In Italy, surgeons at age 65 are obligated to continue working in the healthcare sector rather than retire.

In 2014, Katlic and Coleman discussed the program developed and implemented at Sinai Hospital in Baltimore, designed to evaluate objectively a surgeon's physical and cognitive function.[8] The aging surgeon program is a 2-day comprehensive, multidisciplinary, and objective evaluation of surgeons' cognitive and physical function. The stated goals of the program are protecting surgeons from unreliable assessment of competency or cognitive ability; identifying reversible disorders whose treatment might improve function; aiding surgeons in the decision to retire; protecting patients from unsafe surgeons; protecting surgeon and hospital liability risks, and others.

Sinai Hospital's multidisciplinary team includes experts in neurology, neuropsychology, surgery, physical medicine and rehabilitation, geriatric surgery, internal medicine, ophthalmology, law, and ethics. The program requires a pre-screening medical history. On day one of the program, the surgeon undergoes physical and neurologic examination, a PT/OT (physical therapy and occupational therapy) evaluation of reaction time, fine motor function, coordination, and other parameters, and neuropsychological testing. On day two, additional neuropsychological and PT/OT evaluations are performed, as well as an ophthalmologic evaluation and exit interview.

Medical Musings

The authors stated that the confidential final report includes only objective findings and offers no recommendations regarding surgeon's operating privileges or retirement. The authors stated that the reports are sent in an encrypted, locked electronic file to whomever paid for the program-i.e., surgeon, hospital or chief of surgery. The authors point out that their program balances patient safety and liability risks while maintaining the dignity of the surgeon and his or her value to society. The time for aging physicians to stop practicing due to competency issues remains a current topic in the literature.[44,45]

Reviewing how performance issues have been addressed for pilots provides evidence and suggests strategies that might be applied to physicians. An article by Carroll published in 1992 and sponsored by the Air Force Research Laboratory/RHA War fighter Readiness Research Division (Mesa, Ariz.) discussed situational awareness (SA), its definition, and how to measure it objectively.[46] At the time of that publication Carroll reported that an Air Staff process action team had been created to address these questions. He stated that defining SA had been approached from many directions and resulted in different viewpoints from operators and technicians.

Carroll stated that the Major Command (MAJCOM) training programs did not have a focus on SA. The programs that were in place included: (1) Cockpit Attention Task Management (CATM); (2) Aircrew Attention Awareness Management Program (AAAMP); (3) Cockpit Resource Management (CRM); and (4) Mission Oriented Simulator Training (MOST); and (5) Aircrew Coordination Training Program (ACT). He stated that emphasis had been placed on task management, spatial orientation, gravity-induced loss of consciousness (GLOC) and attention. He described SA as 'appearing more as a collateral issue than a goal' of these programs, and Carroll proposed that 'SA' should be 'the umbrella under which applicable human factors research and training are pursued'. He suggested further that 'human factor should be ordered into a supporting role under SA to support mission accomplishment'.

Carroll opined that an individual pilot's experience and capabilities combine to support and maintain a given level of SA, and that SA is affected by the complexity of the mission, intensity of the threat, and the amount of distraction in and out of the cockpit. He provided the definition of SA that was developed by the Air Staff group as 'a pilot's, or aircrew's continuous perception of self and aircraft in relation to the dynamic environment of flight, threats, and mission, and the ability to forecast, then execute tasks based on that perception'. Moreover, 'it is problem solving in a 3-dimensional spatial relationship complicated by the fourth dimension of time compression where there are inherently too few givens and too many variables'. He stated that SA represents cumulative effects of everything that an individual is and does as related to flight performance.

Carroll stated, 'Since the mission of the Air Force is not to maintain spatial orientation, but to fly, to fight and win', focusing on SA should provide a direction to that end point. Carroll suggested further that SA should be the focus of further research with an emphasis on how to 'define, measure, select for, and train human factors and SA'. These concepts and concerns seem directly applicable to surgeons and their activities and mission.

In 1997, researchers Bell and Waag at the Armstrong Laboratory Aircrew Training Research Division in Mesa, Ariz., used observer rating to assess SA in Tactical Air environments.[47] The authors measured SA in operational fighter squadrons and in multiship air combat simulations. The research focused on 3 issues: pilot's definition of SA, the degree to which pilots can judge their fellow pilots' SA reliably, and whether a relationship exists between their judgments and performance.

For the purpose of their study, the authors used the Air Staff definition as SA as reported by Carroll.[44] They pointed out, however, that other definitions of SA were found in the literature.[48-50] The authors recognized that SA is complex and combines processes, tasks, and linkages between them; and they stressed that it is difficult to separate SA from the aspects of skilled performance that have been used to determine proficiency in combat.

Bell and Waag's research focused on whether pilots could use SA to classify fellow pilots validly. The authors, with the assistance of subject-matter experts (SMEs) and instructor pilots, developed a list of 31 behavioral elements of SA. They divided these 31 behaviors into 8 categories of mission: tactical game plan, tactical employment general, tactical employment-BVR, Tactical employment-WVR, information interpretation, and system operation. They limited their study to mission-ready F-I5C pilots.

Bell and Waag developed 4 separate instruments to measure SA. The first instrument asked the pilots to define SA and, based on their personal definition of SA, to rate the importance of each of the 31 elements of SA using a 6-point Likert Scale. The authors designed 3 Situational Awareness Rating Scales (SARS) with 3 different perspectives; self, peers, and supervisory. Data were collected from 238 pilots from 11 squadrons at 4 different Air Force bases. 206 pilots provided their personal definition of SA. The results showed significant agreement on the definition of SA and the ranking of the 31 elements in terms of importance. The analysis of the peer supervisory SARS showed pilots could classify fellow pilots reliably and that squadron ratings of SA correlated with success of mission in simulated air combat missions. The authors proposed that their measures of SA could be used in a squadron's operational training environment by both peers and supervisors to assist in classifying mission-readiness. Similar strategies seem appropriate for surgeons but have not been explored in depth, so far.

Hardy and Parasuraman at the Catholic University of America reported their comprehensive study of cognition and flight performance in older pilots.[51] The authors reviewed the literature from 1939 to 1996 on cognitive aging studies in pilots which found age-related differences in pilots' perception, motor skills, memory, attention, and problem solving/decision making skills. They reported that the measures being used, flight simulation and accident rates, were minimally predictive of flight performance, and they pointed out that the majority of studies related to pilot cognition and/or flying performance used a cross sectional design rather than longitudinal.

Hardy and Parasuraman suggested that the modernization of highly automated aircraft has resulted in qualitative and quantitative changes in cognitive demand. Moreover, these changes in technology have created different types of 'human error', noting that 50 to 75% of fatal aircraft accidents are due to human error.[52]

Many surgeons also are faced with technical challenges such as image guidance, robotic surgery, limited-access surgery, stereotactic surgery, and other approaches; but these have not been incorporated into a formal evaluation assessment for aging physicians.

Hardy and Parasuraman provided a comprehensive review of the theories of cognitive aging, and the impact of cognitive aging on pilots' flight performance. They noted that these theories were based on cognitive performance of non-pilots, both young and old. Theories they discussed included fluid versus crystallized intelligence, decline in inhibition, reduction in processing resources, cognitive slowing, and disuse or under-utilized cognitive abilities. They also questioned whether laboratory tests (static) of cognitive function are representative of real-work (dynamic) cognitive processes. Hardy and Parasuraman cautioned that simulated (SIM) studies are good in the assessment of flight proficiency, but flight performance is measured better by the number of incidences, violations, and accident rates. The authors suggested that more research is needed and should expand upon the typical measurements of flight performance and cognitive skill. In other words, 'examine higher order age-related differences in domain-dependant knowledge and to link these with pilot flight performance'.

Such considerations make sense for doctors, too. However, waiting for 'incidences, violations, and accident rates is not ideal'. It would be better to find valid predictors before a plane crashes or a patient dies.

Causse et al discussed cognitive aging and flight performance in general aviation pilots.[53] They stated that general aviation pilots are not considered professional pilots and thus are not regulated by the FAA's age 60 (now 65) rule[9]; no age limit is specified. The authors examined how age-related cognition impacts pilot performance and ability to make weather-related decisions. Their study focused on three components: cognitive assessment (executive functioning), age of pilot and years of experience, and flight performance. They reported that cognitive assessment was superior to chronological age in predicting pilots' fight performance due to flight experience and the variability of individual aging effects on cognition. It would not be surprising to find similar results among surgeons, but more research is needed.

An article titled, Aging and Situational Awareness: What Pilot Training can Teach Us was accessed from the Internet (from the site A Cognitive Fitness Blog- for Healthy Aging Brain, published February 13, 2013.[54] The author (or blogger) discusses SA and aging, and what can be learned from pilots' training. Pilots undergo 'SIM' (simulated) testing 2 to 3 times a year in which they are tested under simulated flying conditions to determine the pilot's ability to cope with any emergency. SA is described as a skill essential to a pilot's performance in both noncombat and combat flying. The author/blogger posed the question as to whether other professionals such as doctors, teachers, builders, and more should be tested for 'best practice'.

Assessment of cognitive function

Neuropsychologists specialize in the science and clinical practice of cognitive evaluation and identifying brain-behavior relationships. Neuropsychological assessment involves the testing of multiple areas of cognitive functioning via a battery of tests. This often requires periods of 4 to 6 hours or longer. The purpose of this testing is twofold: to assess for current functional impairments as compared to an appropriate normative sample generally, and to collect ideographic cognitive functioning data against which an individual's future test results might be compared.

While we believe that cognitive assessment of physicians is important, such lengthy testing might not be necessary for every evaluation. Nevertheless, if physicians are to undergo cognitive testing routinely, the evaluation protocol must be not only efficient but also standardized, valid, and reliable. With these considerations in mind, we have attempted to construct a protocol to specifically assess those cognitive functions that we believe to be most important to the efficient practice of medicine in the most efficient manner available, utilizing tests and techniques that are well understood and well validated.

A starting point in determining the most germane cognitive domains was to review the existing neuropsychological literature on physician competency, fitness for duty, and impairment. Domains identified in the research as important include various forms of attention, auditory and visual memory, fluid reasoning, quantitative reasoning, verbal reasoning, verbal fluency, visual-spatial reasoning, and processing speed.[53-57]

Within the auditory and visual memory domains in particular, we have selected tests that assess working memory, short-term memory, and long-term memory. Tests assessing each of these functional cognitive domains are identified below. Our suggestions on how they should be used and studied follows the descriptions of the tests.

Auditory attention and concentration

Wechsler Adult Intelligence Scale[58] - *Digit Span subtest* (<5 minutes) - The digit span subtest asks the examinee to recall and repeat accurately increasingly long strings of digits from memory. It includes three tasks designed to test auditory working memory and attention: (1) a digits forward task, (2) a digits backward task, and (3) a digits sequencing task. The first is a test of simple auditory attention, while the latter two are tests of more complex attention and working memory. Taken as a whole, the subtest has high internal validity, high test-retest reliability, and good sensitivity to attentional and auditory working memory impairments.[59]

Wechsler Adult Intelligence Scale IV Letter-Number Sequencing (<5 minutes) - Similar to the Digit Span subtest, the Letter-Number Sequencing subtest asks examinees to accurately recall, sequence and repeat a string of mixed letters and numbers from memory. It is a test of complex attention, working memory, and mental control. It has high internal validity, high test-retest reliability, and is sensitive to attentional impairments.

Paced Auditory Serial Addition Task (Gronwall version)[60] (<10 minutes) - The PASAT is a challenging task that asks examinees to add mentally the last two digits that they heard spoken and say the sum, while simultaneously listening for and remembering the next digit in the sequence. The digit presentation increases in rapidity over time. It is a test of divided auditory attention, sustained attention, mental arithmetic, working memory, and information processing speed.[61] It is a well-validated test with very high internal validity, adequate to high test-retest reliability and is sensitive to attentional impairments.

Visual attention and concentration

Ruff 2 and 7 (5 minutes)[62,63] - The Ruff 2 and 7 asks examinees to scan quickly and accurately strings of numbers or letters sequentially while marking only the 2s and 7s. It is a test of sustained visual attention, selective attention, and visual discrepancy analysis with high internal validity, adequate to high test-retest reliability, and good sensitivity to attentional impairments.

Symbol Digit Modalities Test[64,65] (Oral and Written Modalities) (3 minutes) - The Symbol Digit Modalities Test asks examinees to quickly and accurately record a series of digits associated with a set of symbols listed in a key at the top of the test form. It includes separate written and verbal recording components. It is a test of divided attention, simple visual attention, and processing speed. It is sensitive to attentional impairments and includes a comparison of processing speed abilities between the oral and written presentations. Test-retest reliability has been found to be somewhat variable, however, and it is known to be sensitive to examinee fatigue.

Auditory/verbal memory (immediate and delayed)

Wechsler Memory Scale[66,67] - *Logical Memory I and Logical Memory II* (<15 minutes) - These tests ask examinees to listen to several stories and then repeat them back verbatim. They measure immediate and delayed recall of complex auditory information. Logical Memory I (immediate recall) has high internal consistency, while Logical Memory II (delayed recall) shows adequate internal consistency. Test-retest reliability for both is somewhat variable. Both show good sensitivity to memory disturbances in a variety of patient populations.

California Verbal Learning Test[68,69] *immediate and delayed recall*) (<20 minutes) - This test asks examinees to listen to a series of words and repeat them back over multiple trials. It measures encoding capacity for auditory information, immediate and delayed recognition of words, retrieval efficacy, learning strategy, acquisition rate, and proactive and retroactive interference. Test-retest reliability is high for overall scores. It is sensitive to memory disturbances in a variety of patient populations.

Visual Memory (working, immediate and delayed)

Wechsler Memory Scale IV[66] - *Symbol Span Test* (<10 minutes) - This test presents examinees with a series of increasingly long sequences of nonsense designs which they are required to recognize and select from a lineup of similar symbols. It tests visual memory span and visual working memory. Performance is scored for correct

selection of symbols in the correct order after a brief presentation. The test has shown good discriminative sensitivity to dementia and brain injury versus normal patients.[70]
Rey-Osterrieth Complex Figures Test[71,72] (8 to 15 minutes). This test briefly presents examinees with a complex 2-dimensional design which they must first copy accurately and then later draw from memory. It assesses visual-spatial constructional ability, as well as immediate and delayed visual memory. Although there are different forms with different scoring systems, it has adequate to high inter-rater and intra-rater reliability for total scores. The cognitive operations required for adequate performance include visual perception, visual-spatial organization, motor functioning and, on the recall conditions, immediate and delayed visual memory. It is a reliable measure of visual-constructional ability (copy phase) and memory (recall phases).

Visual processing speed

Ruff 2 and 7 - see above
Symbol Digit Modalities Test - see above.
Trail Making Test A and B[73] (<5 minutes) - This is a visual scanning, sequencing, and processing speed test consisting of two parts: Part A requires simple scanning and accurate sequencing of letters, while Part B adds an alternating letter-number sequencing component. It is a test of mental flexibility, impulse inhibition, and executive control. Test-retest reliability is adequate with good inter-rater reliability and good sensitivity to attentional impairments.[70]

Auditory and verbal processing speed

Paced Auditory Serial Addition Task (see above).
Controlled Oral Word Association Test <5 minutes) - This test asks examinees to produce spontaneously orally as many words as they can which begin with a certain letter. It has high internal validity, high test-retest reliability, and known sensitivity to traumatic brain injuries, dementing illness, and frontal lobe impairments. Test-retest reliability is good, as is inter-rater reliability.[74-76]
Symbol Digit Modalities Test (see above).

Visual constructional skills

Rey Complex Figure Test (see above).
Clock Drawing Test[77,78] (<2 minutes) - This test asks examinees to draw from memory an analogue clock displaying a specific time. It is a screening measure for visuoperceptual and visuospatial impairments, working memory, and executive and

motor functions. Although there are numerous scoring methods in use, the various protocols tend to be highly correlated with one another. In the dementia and brain injury contexts, this measure shows moderate correlations with measures of temporal orientation, visual-spatial/visual-constructional skill, and with measures of executive functioning. Given its sensitivity and specificity in dementia assessments it is widely used as a quick 'scan' for cognitive impairments in adults.[70]

Quantitative reasoning

Wechsler Adult Intelligence Scale IV[58,59,70] - Arithmetic subtest (<10 minutes) - This test consists of arithmetic problems presented in an auditory story format in order of increasing difficulty, requiring the examinee to discern relevant quantitative information and apply the correct mental calculation to solve a story problem. The task taps mental manipulation, concentration, attention, working and short-term memory, and numerical reasoning. It has been shown to be sensitive to an array of cognitive problems, but is not considered a reliably specific indicator of any one set of cognitive impairments.[79]

Higher level executive functions (multitasking, cognitive flexibility, planning, and problem-solving)

Paced Auditory Serial Addition Task (see above).
Rey Complex Figure Test (see above).
Trail Making Test A and B (see above).
Controlled oral word association test (see above).

Abbreviated Category Test[80] (20 minutes) - This test presents examinees with a visual puzzle and requires them to deduce a numerical solution based on very limited feedback. It measures abstraction or concept formation ability, mental flexibility in the face of complex and novel problem solving, and capacity to learn from experience. This abbreviated version functions in a similar fashion to the full-length version used in the Halstead-Reitan in terms of its psychometric properties and discriminative ability. It has high reliability for samples of normal and brain-damaged adults with variable test-retest reliability. It is sensitive to a variety of brain disturbances and is almost as sensitive as the full Halstead-Reitan Neuropsychological Test Battery[65] in identifying the presence or absence of neurological damage.[70,79,81]

Stroop Test[82,83] (5 minutes) - This test presents mixed written and colored stimuli to examinees and requires them to rapidly read and articulate a controlled, often counter-intuitive response. It measures cognitive control, mental flexibility, and suppression of habitual responses. It has moderate to high internal validity and high test-retest reliability. Its specificity with respect to certain impairments, especially frontal lobe injuries, is high, although its sensitivity is variable.

Conclusion

Assessing performance in aging physicians is important for patient safety. Disciplinary actions occur much more frequently against doctors who have been out of medical school for 40 years than against those who have been out for 10 years.[84] Moreover, performance on various outcomes decline as physicians age.[20] Unfortunately, there appears to be no relationship between an older physicians' assessment of his/her cognitive skills and objective cognitive measures,[37] and older surgeons perform poorly compared with younger surgeons when performing complex operations.[17] Nevertheless, even the most recent efforts by the AMA have failed to result in specific recommendations.[85]

Having valid, reliable objective predictors of performance decrement would be invaluable to those of us responsible for credentialing, to patients, and to aging physicians themselves. While several approaches have been proposed for cognitive assessment of aging physicians, none has been adopted widely. Perhaps more importantly, none has been applied over time to determine whether cognitive abnormalities detected are well compensated issues that have been present for a lifetime or new deficiencies related to aging.

It is also possible that youthful physician performance is at the upper end of the normal range and that 'normal' results at the lower end of normal parameters actually might represent cognitive decline in an aging physician. Longitudinal testing will be needed to establish each physician's baseline function and cognitive stability/change over time, so that more frequent testing during older years can be interpreted meaningfully.

We concur with the suggestion of Richard Homan, MD, (personal communication, November 15, 2015) that performance on competency-based board precertification examinations over time (7- to 10-year intervals) might provide an early warning of decline; and we encourage correlation of the measures that we suggest here with examination performance over a career.

In addition, although there are some data from research on pilots suggesting that cognitive decline correlates with decreased pilots' performance (tested typically with simulators), there few data correlating cognitive changes in physicians directly with deterioration in patient care in the operating room or the office. At present, although cognitive decline is of concern, care should be exercised not to assume that it correlates with clinically significant impairment in physician function (in the operating room, for example) in the absence of evidence. Whether that evidence is obtained by correlating cognitive test results with patient outcomes data, or with physician performance in simulators, we believe that it is essential that the correlations (or lack thereof) be established before cognitive or other test results are used to affect physician privileges.

We believe that the lack of information available in the literature is due to the complexity involved in obtaining valid, reliable and practical data; but we believe that the question is important enough to justify embarking on a multi-year, multi-institutional study of cognitive function (and associated changes), over time, correlated with physician performance and patient outcomes. We have proposed a brief neuropsychological test battery that is still longer than we would like (close to 2 hours, as compared with the 4 to 6 hour routine comprehensive neuropsychological test battery); but we selected the tests in this battery because we believe that it will provide sufficient sensitivity and validity to detect many age-mediated cognitive changes that are potentially relevant across a range of cognitive domains. We offered this proposed protocol for comment and criticism. We hope that the medical and neuropsychological communities can reach a consensus on a cognitive test battery that will be applied widely by multiple institutions so that a large volume of longitudinal data can be acquired during medical student years and continuing throughout the latest decades of life, along with physician performance data collected over time. Such data also are likely to provide evidence that will permit shortening the test battery.

Motor function data have not been addressed in this chapter; but motor assessment is important, especially for surgeons and other physicians who perform procedures. However, motor assessment and its integration with cognitive data into overall physician performance assessment are beyond the scope of this chapter.

This chapter also has not discussed assessment of frailty. Frailty has been used to predict outcomes in our patients[86-88] and requires a relatively simple, quick assessment. To the best of our knowledge, no one has performed frailty assessments on physicians to determine whether increasing frailty correlates with physician performance. Although this topic is also outside the scope of the chapter, we believe that acquiring motor and frailty data simultaneously with cognitive data might be of great value. For example, at present, we have no idea whether a simple frailty assessment might provide all the information that we need in assessing aging physicians. While this seems somewhat unlikely, there is no evidence either way.

We hope that this chapter's call for collaborative research into cognitive changes over time and their functional implications will lead to movement toward consensus on a cognitive test battery, and a national or international collaborative research venture possibly combined with motor and frailty assessments, that eventually will provide the kind of valid, reliable information that is needed to help understand and guide age-related changes in physicians, to optimize physician productivity in the later years of life, and to protect our patients.

References

1. Bunkin IA. When does a surgeon retire? *JAMA* 1983;250(6):757–8.
2. Greenfield LJ, Proctor MC. Attitudes toward retirement: A survey of the American Surgical Association. *Ann Surg* 1994;220(3):387–90.
3. Greenfield LJ. Farewell to surgery. *J Vasc Surg* 1994;19(1):6–14.
4. Stauger R. Boredom on the assembly line: Age and personality variables. *Industrial Gerontology* 1975;30:23–43.
5. Rosen B. Management perceptions of older employees. *Monthly Labor Review* 1978;101(5):33–5.
6. Tzankoff SP, Norris AH. Age-related differences in lactate distribution kinetics following maximal exercise. *Eur J Appl Physiol Occup Physiol* 1979;42(1):35–40.
7. The Age Discrimination in Employment Act of 1967. (Pub. L. No. 90-202, 81 Stat). 602. 1967.
8. Katlic MR, Coleman J. The aging surgeon. *Ann Surg* 2014;260(2):199–201.
9. Federal Register. Federal aviation regulations, Part 121.383 (Doc. No. 6258, 29 FR 191212). 1978.
10. Ripple GP. Federal court: Mandatory retirement age for pilots is not age discrimination. National Business Aviation Association May 2, 2014. Available at: www.nbaa.org/admin/personnel/age-60/20140502-federal-court-mandatory-retirement-age-for-pilots-is-not-age-discrimination.php. Accessed March 9, 2016.
11. Federal Aviation Administration. Pilot age 65 retirement law. FAA statement on pilot retirement age. Available at: www.faa.gov/licenses_certificates/airmen_certification/pilot_age_65. Accessed March 9, 2016.
12. Powell DH, Kaplan EF, Whitla D, et al. *Microcog: Assessment of Cognitive Functioning*. Ver. 2.1. San Antonio, Texas: The Psychological Corporation; 1993.
13. Trunkey DD, Botney R. Assessing competency: A tale of two professions. *J Am Coll Surg* 2001;192(3):385–95.
14. Stewart JB. *Blind Eye: The Terrifying Story of a Doctor Who Got Away with Murder*. New York, New York: Simon and Schuster; 1999:161.

15. Morris W. *American Heritage Dictionary of the English Language*. Boston, Massachusetts: Houghton Mifflin Co; 1981.
16. Howard M. Personal communications. Quantico, Virginia: Federal Bureau of Investigation; cited in Assessing competency: A tale of two professions. *J Am Coll Surg* 2001;192(3):389.
17. Waljee JF, Greenfield LJ, Dimick JB, Birkmeyer JD. Surgeon age and operative mortality in the United States. *Ann Surg* 2006;244(3):353–62.
18. Hummer CD III. The aging surgeon: How old is too old? AAOS Now 2007. Available at: www.aaos.org/news/bulletin/may07/managing4.asp. Accessed March 9, 2016
19. Blasier RB. The problem of the aging surgeon: When surgeon age becomes a surgical risk factor. *Clin Orthop Relat Res* 2009;467(2):402–11.
20. Choudhry NK, Fletcher RH, Soumerai SB. Systematic review: The relationship between clinical experience and quality of health care. *Ann Intern Med* 2005;142(4):260–73.
21. Johnson FE, Novell LA, Coplin MA, et al. How practice patterns in colon cancer patient follow-up are affected by surgeon age. *Surg Oncol* 1996;5(3):127–31.
22. Margenthaler JA, Johnson DY, Virgo KS, et al. Evaluation of patients with clinically suspected melanoma recurrence: Current practice patterns of plastic surgeons. *Int J Oncol* 2002;21(3):591–6.
23. O'Neill L, Lanska DJ, Hartz A. Surgeon characteristics associate with mortality and morbidity following carotid endarterectomy. *Neurology* 2000;55(6):733–81.
24. Ahmad S, Lettsome L. Schuricht A. The role of laparoscopy in the management of groin hernia. *JSLS* 1998;2(2):169–73.
25. Callaghan CJ, Couto E, Kerin MJ, et al. Breast reconstruction in the United Kingdom and Ireland. *Br J Surg* 2002;89(3):335–40.
26. Draper B, Winfield S. Luscombe G. The older psychiatrist and retirement. *Int J Geriatr Psychiatry* 1997;12(2):233–9.
27. Greenfield LJ, Proctor MC. When should a surgeon retire? *Adv Surg* 1999;32:385–93.
28. Heck DA, Robinson RL, Partridge CM, et al. Patient outcomes after knee replacement. *Clin Orthop Relat Res* 1998;356:93–110.
29. Neumayer LA, Gawande AA, Wang J, et al. Proficiency of surgeons in inguinal hernia repair: Effect of experience and age. *Ann Surg* 2005;242(3):344–48; discussion 348–52.
30. Rovit RL. To everything there is a season and a time to every purpose: Retirement and the neurosurgeon. *J Neurosug* 2004;100(6):1123-9.

31. The Employment Equality (Age) Regulations 2006. CompactLaw. Available at: www.compactlaw.co.uk/free-legal-articles/age-discrimination.html. Accessed March 9, 2016.
32. Retirement age.GOV.UK. Updated Feb. 5, 2016. Available at: www.gov.uk/retirement-age. Accessed March 9, 2016.
33. AgeDiscrimination.info. The finalized Employment Equality (Repeal of Retirement Age Provisions) Regulations 2011 are now out.March 4, 2011. Available at: www.agediscrimination.info/Pages/ItemPage.aspx?Item=353. Accessed March 9, 2016.
34. Boom-Saad Z, Langenecker SA, Bieliauskas LA, et al. Surgeons outperform normative controls on neuropsychologic tests, but age-related decay of skills persists. *Am J Surg* 2008;195(2):205–9.
35. Robbins TW, James M, Owen AM, et al. A study of performance on tests from the CANTAB battery sensitive to frontal lobe dysfunction in a large sample of normal volunteers: Implications for theories of executive functioning and cognitive aging. Cambridge Neuropsychological Test Automated Battery. *J Int Neuropsychol Soc* 1998;4 (5):474–90.
36. Sahakian BJ, Owen AM. Computerized assessment in neuropsychiatry using CANTAB: Discussion paper. *J R Soc Med* 1992; 85(7):399–402.
37. Bieliauskas LA, Langenecker S, Graver C, et al. Cognitive changes and retirement among senior surgeons (CCRASS); Results from the CCRASS study. *J Am Coll Surg* 2008;207 (1):69–78.
38. Drag LL, Bieliauskas LA, Langenecker SA, Greenfield LJ. Cognitive functioning, retirement status, and age: Results from the Cognitive Changes and Retirement among Senior Surgeons study. *J Am Coll Surg* 2010;211(3):303–7.
39. Carmel PW. Senior physicians keep working, putting off the R-word. American Medical News. April 30, 2012. Available at: www.amednews.com/article/20120430/opinion/304309967/5/. Accessed March 9, 2016.
40. Tarkan L. As doctors age, worries about their ability grow. *The New York Times*. January 24, 2011. Available at: www.nytimes.com/2011/01/25/health/25doctors.html?_r=2&ref=science&. Accessed March 9, 2016.
41. Garrett K, Kaups KL. The aging surgeon: When is it time to leave active practice? *Bull Am Coll Surg* 2014;99(4):32–5.
42. Stanford J. New policy to require evaluations for late-career practitioners. Inside Stanford Medicine.July 16, 2012. Available at: https://med.stanford.edu/news/all-news/2012/07/new-policy-to-require-evaluations-for-late-career-practitioners.html. Accessed March 9, 2016.

43. Sun GH. Clinicians are talking about aging surgeons. Medscape Family Medicine.July 21, 2014. Available at: www.medscape.com/viewarticle/828329. Accessed March 9, 2016.
44. Tanner L. Aging MDs prompt call for competency tests at AMA meeting. Washington's Top News.June 8, 2015. Available at: wtop.com/health/2015/06/aging-mds-prompt-call-for-competency-tests-at-ama-meeting/. Accessed March 9, 2016.
45. Holt GR. Age of surgeons may raise ethical concerns over memory lapses. ENT Today.August 11, 2015. Available at: www.enttoday.org/article/age-of-surgeons-may-raise-ethical-concerns-over-memory-lapses/2/?singlepage=1. Accessed March 9, 2016.
46. Carroll LA. Desperately seeking SA. TAG Attack ;(TAG SP 127-1) 1992:32:5–6.
47. Bell HH, Waag WL. Using observer ratings to assess situational awareness in tactical air environments. United States Air Force Armstrong Laboratory, Mesa, Ariz; March 1997. Available at: www.dtic.mil/dtic/tr/fulltext/u2/a459801.pdf. Accessed March 9, 2016.
48. Endsley MR. Toward a theory of situation awareness in dynamic systems. *Hum Factors* 1995:37(1):32–64.
49. Sarter NB, Woods DD. Situation awareness: A critical but ill-defined phenomenon. *Int J Aviation Psychol* 1991;1(1):45–57.
50. Tenney YJ, Adams MJ, Pew RW, et al. A principled approach to the measurement of situation awareness in commercial aviation.NASA Contractor Report 4451. Available at: http://ntrs.nasa.gov/archive/nasa/casi.ntrs.nasa.gov/19920021063.pdf. Accessed March 9, 2016.
51. Hardy D, Parasurman R. Cognition and flight performance in older pilots. *J Exper Psychol Appl* 1997;3(4):313–48.
52. Baker SP, Lamb MW, Li G, Dodd RS. Human factors in crashes of commuter airplanes. *Aviat Space Environ Med* 1993;64(1):63–8.
53. Causse M, Dehais F, Arexis M, Pastor J. Cognitive aging and flight performances in general aviation pilots. *Neuropsychol Dev Cogn B Aging Neuropscychol Cogn* 2011;18(5):544–61.
54. M Margaret. Aging and situational awareness: What pilot training can teach us. A Cognitive Fitness Blog-for a healthy aging brain. February 13, 2014. Available at: http://mybrainfitness.wordpress.com/2013/02/13/aging-and-situational-awareness-what-pilot-training-can-teach-us-2/. Accessed March 9, 2016.

55. Korinek LL, Thompson LL, McRae C, Korinek E. Do physicians referred for competency evaluations have underlying cognitive problems? *Acad Med* 2009;84(8):1015–21.
56. Turnbull J, Cunnington J, Unsal A, et al. Competence and cognitive difficulty in physicians: A follow-up study. *Acad Med* 2006;81(10):915–18.
57. Perry W, Crean RD. A retrospective review of the neuropsychological test performance of physicians referred for medical infractions *Arch Clin Neuropsychol* 2005;20(2):161–70.
58. Wechsler D. *Wechsler Adult Intelligence Scale-4th Edition Test Manual*. San Antonio, Texas: Pearson; 2008.
59. Kaplan E, Fein D, Morris R, Delis D. *WAIS-R as a Neuropsychological Instrument*. San Antonio, Texas: The Psychological Corporation; 1991.
60. Gronwall DM. Paced Auditory Serial-Addition Task: A measure of recovery from concussion. *Percept Mot Skills* 1977;44(2):367–73.
61. Crawford JR, Obonsawin MC, Allen KM. PASAT and components of WAIS-R performance: Convergent and discriminant validity. *Neuropsycholog Rehab* 1998;8(3):255–72.
62. Ruff RM, Allen CC. *Ruff 2 and 7 Selective Attention Test*. Odessa, Florida: Psychological Assessment Resources, Inc.; 1996.
63. Ruff RM, Niemann H, Allen CC, et al. The Ruff 2 and 7 Selective Attention Test: A neuropsychological application *Percept Mot Skills* 1992;75(3 Pt 2):1311–19.
64. Smith A. *Symbol Digit Modalities Test Manual* (revised). Los Angeles, California: Western Psychological Services; 1982.
65. Shum DH, McFarland KA, Bain JD. Construct validity of eight tests of attention: Comparison of normal and closed head injured samples. *Clin Neuropsychol* 1990;4(2):151–62.
66. Wechsler D. *Wechsler Memory Scale-4th Edition Test Manual*. San Antonio, Texas: Pearson; 2009.
67. Ryan JJ, Ament PA, Arb JD. Supplementary WMS-III tables for determining primary subtest strengths and weaknesses. *Psycholog Assess* 2000;12:193–6.
68. Delis DC, Kramer JH, Kaplan E, Ober BA. California Verbal Learning Test - 2nd Edition. San Antonio, Texas: Psychological Corporation; 2000.
69. Woods SP, Delis DC, Scott JC, et al. The California Verbal Learning Test-second edition: Test-retest reliability, practice effects, and reliable change indices for the standard and alternate forms. *Arch Clin Neuropsychol* 2006;21(5):413–20.
70. Lezak MD, Howieson DB, Bigler ED, Tranel D. *Neuropsychological Assessment*. 5th ed. New York, New York: Oxford University Press; 2012.

71. Osterrieth PA. Le test de copie d'une figure complexe, *Archives De Psychologie* 1944; 30:206–356 [translated by Corwin J, Bylema PW]. *Clin Neuropsychol* 1993;7:9–15.
72. Baser CA, Ruff RM. Construct validity of the San Diego Neuropsychological Test Battery. *Arch Clin Neuropsychol* 1987;2(1):13–32.
73. Reitan RM. Validity of the Trail Making Test as an indicator of organic brain damage. *Percept Mot Skills* 1958;8:271–6.
74. Benton A, Hamsher K, Sivan A. *Multilingual Aphasia Examination*. 3rd ed. Lutz, Florida: Psychological Assessment Resources; 1994.
75. Henry JD, Crawford JR. A meta-analytic review of verbal fluency performance in patients following focal cortical lesions. *Neuropsychology* 2004;18(2):284–95.
76. Henry JD, Crawford JR. A meta-analytic review of verbal fluency performance in patients with traumatic brain injury. *Neuropsychology* 2004;18(4):621–8.
77. Borod JC, Goodglass H, Kaplan E. Normative data on the Boston Diagnostic Aphasia Examination, Parietal Lobe Battery, and the Boston Naming Test. *J Clin Neuropsychol* 1980;2:209–15.
78. Freedman M, Leach L, Kaplan E, et al. *Clock drawing: A Neuropsychological Analysis*. New York, New York: Oxford University Press; 1994.
79. Mitrushina M, Boone KB, Razani J, D'Elia LF. *Handbook of Normative Data for Neuropsychological Assessment*. 2nd ed. New York, New York: Oxford University Press; 2005.
80. Charter RA, Swift KM, Blusewicz MJ. Age- and education-corrected standardized short form of the Category Test. *Clin Neuropsychol* 1997;11:142–5.
81. DeFilippis NA, McCampbell E. *Booklet Category Test*. 2nd ed. Odessa, Florida: Psychological Assessment Resources; 1997.
82. Dodrill CB. A neuropsychological battery for epilepsy. *Epilepsia* 1978;19(6):611–23.
83. Strauss E, Sherman EM, Spreen O. *A Compendium of Neuropsychological Tests: Administration, Norms, and Commentary*. 3rd ed. New York, New York: Oxford University Press; 2006.
84. Khaliq AA, Dimassi H, Huang CY, et al. Diciplinary action against physicians: Who is likely to get disciplined? *Am J Med* 2005;118(7):773–7.
85. Paige L. Should older physicians be tested for competence at age 65? Available at: www.medscapee.com/viewarticle/848937. October 28, 2015. Accessed March 9, 2016.

86. Raghunandan V, Maegawa FB. Frailty index predicts the risk of morbidity and mortality after pancreaticoduodenectomy-an NSQIP study. *J Am Coll Surg* 2015;221(4):S81–2.
87. Raghunandan V, Maegawa FB. Frailty is a predictor of adverse outcomes after hepatic resections for hepatocellular carcinoma. *J Am Coll Surg* 2015;221(4):S82.
88. Robinson TN, Waltson JD, Brummel NE, et al. Frailty for surgeons: Review of a National Institute on Aging conference on frailty for specialists. *J Am Coll Surg* 2015; 221(6):1083–92.

Reprinted with modifications by permission of Vendome Group from:

Sataloff, RT, Hawkshaw MJ, Maitz E, Kutinsky J. The aging physician and surgeon. *ENT J* 2016;95(4,5):E35–48.

Part VI: Miscellaneous Musings

56. Teamwork

Healthcare team collaboration has been key to numerous developments in medicine. Physicians have advanced their subspecialties through assembling teams, without which some of our most notable successes might not have been possible. For example, extensive, complex skull base surgery requires close collaboration among otologists, head and neck surgeons, neurosurgeons, anesthesiologists, intensivists, oncologists, radiation oncologists, nurses, psychological professionals, social workers, nutritionists, and others. State-of-the-art in professional voice care and the evolution of the subspecialty of laryngology were dependent upon voice teams, including laryngologists, speech-language pathologists, singing voice specialists, voice scientists, acting voice specialists, nurses, anesthesiologists, pulmonologists, neurologists, gastroenterologists, and others.

For some professionals, interdisciplinary collaboration and teamwork come naturally. For others, the concept sounds good, but execution can be challenging. This may be true particularly for traditional surgeons who are accustomed to working alone, 'running the show', and having total control. Recognizing the importance of teamwork and the intricacies of establishing and maintaining a successful team, the American College of Surgeons (ACS) convened an ad hoc committee and developed a 'Statement on high performance teams' that was approved by the Board of Regents of the ACS in October 2009. The brief statement is insightful, and all physicians would benefit from considering its precepts. Although the statement was directed primarily at surgical teams, it is equally applicable to team collaborations in other venues.

The ACS statement has crystallized critical attributes of high-performing teams. These include:

- A commitment by all team members to teamwork for the best interest of the patient
- Respectful behaviors, where contributions of all disciplines and providers are valued
- Recognition and constructive resolution of conflict
- Coordination among all team members that includes accountability for mutual performance awareness and backup behaviors
- Leadership characterized by:
  - ☐ Clearly defined leadership roles
  - ☐ Leadership style appropriate to the clinical situation
  - ☐ Clear direction to the team
  - ☐ Continuous solicitation of input from team members, and team-based decision making
- Timely, accurate, and structured communication with verification of understanding
- Effective care coordination, including structured hand-offs through all phases of care
- Ability to remain flexible and adaptable to changing situations

These 'critical attributes' are well conceived, but they are not as simple to achieve as they might seem. Leadership styles of high-power surgical professionals are not always optimally sensitive to the needs of other team members, particularly non-surgeon (or non-physician) colleagues. In addition, leadership of a team also requires the ability to follow, and to listen with a truly open mind to input from other members of the team. One of the great benefits of teamwork is the collaboration of people who have expertise in different (but overlapping) areas. A good leader has to have as much intuitive respect for the knowledge and importance of each member of the team as for his/her own contribution and knowledge. Also, it is easy to talk about communication, and few would argue against its importance; but it requires time that many of us do not have. In order for a team to function as it should, every member of the team (including the physician) has to make it a priority to take the time to interact effectively and communicate with other team members.

The ACS statement also addresses obligations of healthcare organizations and lists 'four critical components for success':

- Ensuring that all staff learn and use team-based knowledge, skills, and attitudes (the institution must provide appropriate education and training)

- Providing opportunities to practice team-based skills in a supportive environment that includes feedback and fosters experiential learning
- Building teamwork techniques, prompts, and structure into the institutional workflow, such that teamwork becomes the routine and team behaviors are the norm
- Institutional leadership and governance must support sustained team-based practice through the following:
  - ☐ Recurrent refresher training
  - ☐ Monitoring performance
  - ☐ Rewards for teamwork and team behaviors
  - ☐ Willingness to sanction noncompliant individuals regardless of status or role

The ACS's Ad Hoc Committee on the Development of High Performance Teamwork in Surgery Through Education should be commended. Its statement, the essence of which is included in this chapter (with minor modifications and omissions), crystallizes the elements needed for successful collaboration. The guidelines embrace intellectual open-mindedness, appropriate behavior, and efficient communication. Teams that incorporate these principles successfully not only provide state-of-the-art patient care, but they also advance our knowledge through interdisciplinary intellectual creativity.

When teamwork functions at its best, the whole truly is greater than the sum of the parts. All physicians should benefit from consideration of these principles, whether they are collaborating in a quaternary clinical care team, or simply trying to optimize a team to make an office run well. The teamwork concepts are universal, but that does not mean that they happen without thought, work, ongoing assessment, and constant change.

Reprinted with modifications by permission of Vendome Group from:
Sataloff RT. Teamwork. *ENT J* 2010;89(5):206–7.

57. Longevity: The disposable soma?

From the first alchemist's elixir of life to J.K. Rowling's *Harry Potter and the Sorcerer's Stone*, people have fantasized about immortality. Strictly speaking, one might argue that the body needs to exist only long enough to procreate. The soma (all of the body's cells except for the sex cells) is disposable once genes have been passed to the next generation. Nevertheless, the human desire for somatic survival, coupled with scientific development, has resulted in an ever-lengthening human life span. It is interesting to consider whether we are getting closer to an indefinitely lengthened life span.

While most of us have considered death inevitable, is that presumption a scientific certainty? People age and die by having their components wear out and break down. If we were cars, those parts could be replaced, and we might be kept on the road almost indefinitely. Aging science (and philosophy) might be moving us closer and closer to the point at which our bodily destruction can be delayed, prevented, or even repaired.

One controversial, visionary proponent of anti-aging technology is Aubrey de Grey, PhD. He is editor-in-chief of the peer-reviewed academic *journal Rejuvenation Research*, which publishes articles on aging intervention. Dr. de Grey has published widely, and his writings include an interesting book written for the general public entitled Ending Aging: The Rejuvenation Breakthroughs That Could Reverse Human Aging in Our Lifetime that provides an overview of aging science.[1] Dr. de Grey is an engineer, and his biotechnologic vision of aging is interesting and provocative, if somewhat troublesome for traditional biologists.

Dr. de Grey has developed Strategies for Engineered Negligible Senescence (SENS). With his engineer's eye, he has divided aging into seven components: cell loss, apoptosis-resistance (the tendency of cells to resist dying when they are supposed to die), gene mutation in the cell nucleus, gene mutation in the mitochondria, the accumulation of 'junk' inside cells, the accumulation of 'junk' outside cells, and the accumulation of inappropriate chemical links in the material that supports cells.[1] While the challenges of defeating aging are formidable, this divides the problem into distinct components that do not seem quite so daunting.

The two primary approaches to these problems are to ameliorate and slow the normal wear and tear, masking its consequences, or to 'service' the body at regular intervals to replace parts that have worn out. Oxidation is a common factor in the final five items on de Grey's list of the seven components of aging. Mainstream science recognizes that mitochondria are important in bodily wear and tear. Sugars are broken down in mitochondria, where they react with oxygen and release energy into cells. They also produce free radicals that oxidize other molecules, including DNA and proteins, causing damage.

There has been extensive research on the use of antioxidants to combat free radicals and slow the process of bodily damage, and other concomitants of aging. Whether one addresses oxidative injury through newly developed antioxidants, vitamins, diet modification, or other means, the importance of addressing oxidative injury is established for a variety of disease states, including some cancers. Its suspected contribution to the aging process does not seem farfetched.

Replacing worn-out parts also is not inconceivable science fiction. Stemcell research has already demonstrated that stem cells may develop into virtually any body component. It is likely that science will learn how to harness, direct, and utilize the potential of stem cells to repair disease or injury. For example, in otolaryngology, there has been discussion about using stem cells to regenerate the superficial layer of lamina propria of vocal folds to treat patients with vocal fold scar and to regenerate inner ear hair cells to reverse deafness. It is quite conceivable that stem-cell science, or as yet unforeseen similar developments, eventually will permit us to repair or replace worn-out bodily cells and organs.

There are other interesting approaches to address aging. For example, one is to find a way to overcome the Hayflick limit on cell reproduction. The Hayflick limit, named after Leonard Hayflick, is the limit on the number of times a given cell can divide. While this varies among species, once the cell reaches its Hayflick limit, it stops dividing (except for stem cells, which do not have a Hayflick limit). The problem with overcoming the Hayflick limit and getting cells to start dividing again is that the process sounds a lot like cancer, and researchers worry (quite reasonably) that malignancy might result from this approach.

Another strategy is starvation. For reasons that are not clear, decreased dietary intake prolongs life. Unfortunately, starvation also has undesirable consequences, such as shutting down ovulation, since survival trumps reproduction as a biological priority. If the body could be led to think it is experiencing the beneficial effects of starvation without actually starving, that might be another approach to increasing longevity. Such manipulation might involve the genes for sirtuins, for example, which are proteins that have been shown to extend life in organisms simpler than humans.

The likelihood of our living indefinitely is low. However, while we physicians are busy combating aging through cosmetic surgery, and other interventions, it behooves us to recognize that there are scientists who dedicate their careers to the problems of aging, and there are provocative thinkers such as Aubrey de Grey who challenge us to hypothesize that aging changes and the disposability of the soma can be overcome. Adopting that hypothesis might lead to interesting and creative research.

Dr. de Grey is one of the few researchers who believes that there are some people currently living who might see their lives extended indefinitely. He bases that extraordinary concept on the hope that further discoveries in life-extending technologies will be made before all of us die, a journey that he refers to as achieving 'longevity escape velocity'. While de Grey's pronouncements seem fantastic, considering them as possible and might be an interesting inspiration to research. Certainly, accepting that 'death is inevitable' is not likely to inspire us to think outside the box. However, believing that death is not inevitable might lead us to develop creative approaches to address aging, longevity and, immortality - topics that should be fascinating to us all.

References

1. de Grey A. *Ending Aging: The Rejuvenation Breakthroughs That Could Reverse Human Aging in Our Lifetime.* New York, New York: St. Martin's Griffin; 2007.

Reprinted with modifications by permission of Vendome Group from:
Sataloff RT. Longevity: The disposable soma? *ENT J* 2010;89(1):8–10.

58. The physician as an expert witness

Physicians practicing in the United States can expect to be involved in medical/legal issues at some time during their careers. Those practicing in 'high-risk' areas might have to address medical/legal issues weekly, if not daily. In addition to trying to protect ourselves from becoming defendants in malpractice litigation, physicians are called upon frequently to serve as expert witnesses, to defend other physicians or on behalf of plaintiffs who are suing physicians. Some physicians refuse to serve as experts under any circumstances, and many are willing to serve only on behalf of the defense. Many have suggested that these approaches are shortsighted.

Reviewing cases (defense or plaintiff) dispassionately to provide opinions based on our best medical judgment is important. If physicians are not willing to review cases (even for the plaintiff), the cases will not simply disappear. Attorneys will find physicians in some specialty (not necessarily with expertise in the subject of the case) with less expertise who will be willing to testify against our colleagues. In many instances, those cases may lack merit. The physicians who take them may not care or, perhaps more commonly, they simply do not have the expertise to recognize that the cases are without merit. Reviewing cases for a good plaintiffs' attorney is important so that he/ she will know when a case lacks merit and will not pursue it. It is also important because it makes us part of the extended process of reviewing our peers and acknowledging bad medical practice (particularly habitually bad medical practice) when it occurs. If we do not participate in ensuring optimal quality within our specialties using every means at our disposal, others will.

If we are going to collaborate with the legal system by serving as expert witnesses, physicians should recognize that there are standards to guide our behavior. Many of us follow the policies established by the American College of Surgeons (ACS), revised in 2007 and approved by the Board of Regents in that year.[1] The statement of the ACS incorporates guidelines promulgated by several other medical groups, including the Council of Medical Specialty Societies. The physician testifying as an expert witness should be aware of the qualifications recommended by the ACS and, in my opinion, should comply with them. These include:

1. The expert witness should have an unrestricted medical license at the time of the occurrence of the event under litigation.
2. The witness should be board-certified by a specialty board recognized by the American Board of Medical Specialties at the time of the incident and qualified in the subject of the case.
3. The specialty of the expert witness should be appropriate to the subject matter in the case.
4. The expert witness should have held privileges to perform the surgical procedure(s) (in a case involving a surgical procedure) in a hospital accredited by The Joint Commission or the American Osteopathic Association, at the time of the incident under litigation.
5. The expert witness should be familiar with the standard of care at the time of the occurrence and should have been involved actively in the clinical practice of the specialty or the subject matter of the case when the incident occurred.
6. The expert witness should have maintained continuing education relative to the specialty or subject matter of the case.
7. The expert witness should be prepared to document the percentage of his/her time involved in serving as an expert witness, as well as the total number of times he/she has testified for the plaintiff or the defendant and his/her fees or compensation.

The ACS also established seven guidelines for the behavior of physicians acting as expert witnesses. These include:

1. Physicians have an obligation to testify in court as expert witnesses when appropriate, and the testimony must be impartial.
2. The physician should review all relevant information, testify to its contents (fairly, honestly, and in a balanced manner), and draw fair and honest conclusions.
3. The expert should distinguish between negligence and unfortunate outcome.

4. The expert should know the standards of practice prevailing at the time and under the circumstances of the incident.
5. The expert witness should be prepared to state the basis of his/her testimony or opinion and to discuss alternate methods and views.
6. Expert witness compensation should be reasonable and commensurate with time and effort. 'It is unethical for a physician expert witness to link compensation to the outcome of a case.'[1]
7. The physician expert witness 'is ethically and legally obligated to tell the truth.'[1] Transcripts of depositions and courtroom testimony are public records and are subject to peer-review. Failure to provide truthful testimony may expose the expert witness to criminal prosecution for perjury, civil suits, and revocation or suspension of his/ her medical license.

All physicians are (hopefully) concerned with quality of care, patient safety, and optimal outcomes, not only for a specific patient and physician, but more broadly for the entire patient population. Whether we like it or not, medical malpractice litigation is one of the methods currently in use to help ensure compliance with standards of practice. We are obligated to review cases involving alleged negligence. During the process, it is important for us to adhere to national standards for qualifications and behavior of expert witnesses, and to provide thoughtful, knowledgeable, and unbiased opinions. Doing so will result in fewer unjustified lawsuits, hopefully fair and reasonable compensation for patients who have been injured avoidably and, ultimately, improvement in patient care.

References

1. Statement on the physician acting as an expert witness. *Bull Am Coll Surg* 2007;92(12):24–5.

Reprinted with modifications by permission of Vendome Group from:
    Sataloff RT. The otolaryngologist as an expert witness. *ENT J* 2009;88(8): 1020–22.

59. Unethical Surgery

On February 6, 2019, the Guardian newspaper (England) published a troubling account of unethical surgery.[1] Although it highlighted the call for retraction of over 400 scientific papers that had been published based on unethical surgery, this issue strikes much deeper than journal publication ethics.

The unusual and insightful article that led to the Guardian coverage was written by Wendy Rogers, a professor of clinical ethics at Macquarie University in Sydney, Australia, and it was published in the well-respected British Medical Journal Open.[2] Rogers reviewed statistics and literature that suggest strongly that a large volume of organ transplant surgery performed in China and reported in English utilized organs obtained unethically from Chinese prisoners. This problem has surfaced before. In 2016, Kilgour et al. published a report documenting an extraordinary discrepancy between the official transplant figures from the Chinese government, and the number of transplants that Chinese hospitals had reported.[3] While the government admitted to 10,000 transplants each year, data from hospitals showed that between 60,000 and 100,000 organs had been transplanted annually. This exceeded by far the number of voluntary organs available, and the evidence suggested that the discrepancy had been filled by organs harvested from prisoners of conscience who had been executed. The European parliament passed a declaration in 2017 that condemned the harvesting of organs from prisoners of conscience, and the parliament had extended a call to the Chinese government to end the practice.

Rogers et al. reviewed all papers published between January 2000 and April 2017 in medical journals published in English that reported on Chinese transplant recipients. Of the 445 studies involving 85,477 transplant patients that they reviewed, only 1% reported whether organ donors had consented to organ donation for transplantation. Disturbingly, the 19 studies that claimed that no organs from executed prisoners had been used occurred prior to 2010; and at that time, there was no volunteer donor program in China. Rogers et al. called for the retraction of more than 400 papers that they believed had utilized organs harvested unethically. The authors argued that journals that publish papers reporting research using organs from executed prisoners are complicit in the unethical conduct. They called for not only immediate retraction of all papers reporting research using organs obtained in this fashion, but also for an international summit to establish policy for "handling Chinese transplant research." They also stressed that having ethics guidelines is insufficient unless they are actually implemented.

In my opinion, the issue is not so much the more than 400 English-language papers that have reported this research (which may be scientifically valid, given the large numbers of transplant operations that have been performed because of the almost unlimited supply of viable organs). The bigger problem is the probability that people are being executed as "prisoners of conscience" so that their organs can be supplied to a willing surgical community and patient population. Western nations have relatively little political control over nations in the Far East, Middle East and elsewhere. Moreover, it is reasonable to argue that we should be very cautious about imposing our values, ethics, and definitions of right and wrong on other nations and other cultures. Nevertheless, lines must be drawn somewhere; and this seems to be a place worth considering, especially since Western science can be considered complicit in this ethical breach. It is no coincidence that those 445 studies were published in English-language journals. Those journals are regarded throughout the world as preeminent, and they establish credibility for the authors who are fortunate enough to have papers accepted in the world's premier journals. If editors and editorial boards had been more vigilant and demanding, those papers would have been rejected, just as we reject out of hand papers reporting human research that do not have institutional review board (IRB) approval. Rogers et al. are quite right. This profound violation of ethics spreads guilt not only among the surgeons and government in China, but also among the editors and publishers who enabled their continued unethical practice by dignifying and validating their activities through publication.

While this situation is extensive, extraordinary and appalling, it also raises questions about what other ethical violations may be getting published "under the radar" and harming segments of the public. This stunning revelation should be a wakeup call for all physicians and especially medical journal editors to examine our specialties, our clinical activities, and the rigor of our journal screening processes in great detail and to avoid diligently any similar ethical violations in all fields of medicine. It also should alert the general population to read medical research critically, even when it is published in the most elite journals.

References

1. Davey, M. Call for retraction of 400 scientific papers amid fears organs came from Chinese prisoners. *The Guardian* February 6, 2019. https://www.theguardian.com/science/2019/feb/06/call-for-retraction-of-400-scientific-papers-amid-fears-organs-came-from-chinese-prisoners. Accessed February 7, 2019.
2. Rogers W, Robertson MP, Ballantyne A, et al. Compliance with ethical standards in the reporting of donor sources and ethics review in peer-reviewed publications involving organ transplantation in China: a scoping review. *BMJ Open* 2019;9(2):e024473. doi:10.1136/bmjopen-2018-024473
3. Kilgar D, Gutmann E, Matas D. Bloody Harvest/The Slaughter: An Update. The International Coalition to End Transplant Abuse. April 30, 2017. https://endtransplantabuse.org/wp-content/uploads/2017/05/Bloody_Harvest-The_Slaughter-2016-Update-V3-and-Addendum-20170430.pdf. Accessed February 7, 2017.

60. Physicians and retirement

In 1905, Sir William Osler famously talked about the "comparative uselessness" of men [*if there had been more than a few women in medicine at the time, he surely would have included them*] older than 40 years and recommended retirement at age 60.[1] Dr. Osler was 55 at the time. It has been established convincingly that although crystallized intelligence remains fairly stable as we age, a decline in fluid intelligence begins during middle age.[2] However, the timing and degree of cognitive decline vary greatly among people. Unfortunately, there are no good metrics to provide evidence-based guidance on when physicians should retire for cognitive reasons, although an approach to developing such information has been proposed.[3] It has been established that there is no relationship between an older physician's self assessment and objective measures of cognitive function.[5] It also has been established that older physicians tend to rely on first clinical impressions based on their experience, rather than on extensive testing;[4] but this tendency contributes to incomplete histories and data acquisition, faulty interpretation, deficient hypotheses and diagnostic error,[6] and jeopardizes patient care.

Retirement is important to all of us. Some of us are approaching "that age." Other doctors practice with "senior" associates. So, issues of aging affect everyone practicing medicine; and they may affect our patients if aging issues are not handled well. That does not just mean ending the practice of older physicians before they start to make medical errors. It also means preparing transition strategies for physicians, practices/departments and health systems. This issue is going to become more pressing. In

1950, 8% of the population of the United States was age 65 or older. In 2000, it was 12%; and by 2050, the number is expected to reach 20%. Life expectancy for males born now is 78 years (1/20 will live past 100); and for females it is 81.2 years (with 1/10 living past 100).[7]

There are many publications on physician retirement and retirement planning, but one of the most helpful is a systematic review by Silver et al. published in 2016.[8] They evaluated 65 English-language articles published between 1978 and 2015. Thirty-three came from the United States, and 32 had been published elsewhere. Their review crystallized a great deal of interesting information.

For example, in 1997, a 50-year-old was expected to work for 13 more years. In 2009, a 50-year-old was expected to work for 16 more years, until age 66. Physicians report that they expect to retire at age 60, but they actually retire at age 69 (three years later than the general population). Mean planned retirement age for otolaryngologists is 67 years,[9] although current convincing data on otolaryngologists' actual retirement age are not available. However, data are available for the years 1996 to 2000; and otolaryngologists in the southeastern United States during that time period retired at 63.5 years of age.[10]

Many factors affect retirement in general. These include increasing lifespan, concerns about the sustainability of social security, and economic market fluctuations. Market fluctuations are especially important for physicians, many of whom have been in private practice and do not have pensions provided by an employer.

Several factors have been identified that influence delay in retirement among physicians. These include flexibility of work hours, intensity of work hours, work satisfaction, other career opportunities (or lack thereof), resource adequacy, sense of intrinsic self-worth, convenience, financial incentives, relationships with co-workers, length of training and late entry into the workforce; attachment to work and related strong work identity, and the 4% rule. The 4% rule says that a person will need approximately 25 times his/her annual expenses in savings/investments in order to retire with a comfortable lifestyle over a 30-year period (anticipating that investments will yield 4% per year). For many physicians, it is difficult to save enough money to afford to retire comfortably using this equation; and the 4% rule can be affected adversely by substantial market downturns, and by longevity greater than 30 years.

There also are factors that influence early retirement among physicians. They include work dissatisfaction, inflexibility, bureaucracy, electronic medical records, burnout, and desire for personal time. Gender is not a major factor. Other issues that figure into retirement timing include cognitive decline, physical decline, dexterity, frailty, and increased error rate (sometimes related to over-reliance on first clinical impressions as noted above). Hence, experience can be an asset or a deterrent.

If physicians remain thorough, diligent and energetic, then experience should be beneficial. However, when physicians start relying on impressions at the expense of comprehensive evaluation, then problems arise.

Physicians are a microcosm of the general public. By 2026, it has been estimated that about 20% of physicians (Canadian) will be 65 or older.[11] In the general population 65 and older, 13% have dementia, and 10% to 20% have at least mild cognitive impairment.[12,13] Studies reviewed by Silver et al. suggest that more than a third of physicians with concerns about competency have mild-to-moderate cognitive impairment.

What needs to be taken into account for retirement planning to be successful? The importance of finances is obvious. Sadly, it is not uncommon for physicians to be unable to afford to retire and maintain a lifestyle that they find acceptable. Physical changes also are important. Physical deterioration can impair not only medical practice, but also the ability to enjoy an active life following retirement. The impact of the psychosocial dynamic of retiring from medical practice should not be underestimated. Much of the identity of many physicians is based in what they do and with whom they work. If physicians have developed no substitute and leave active practice for empty days, dissatisfaction (or worse) may result. Hence, it is helpful to plan a transition to retirement, and perhaps to make it gradual. Practices, institutions and other physician-employment organizations can help this process; and they should be motivated to do so. Organizations benefit from allowing flexibility (change in hours worked, number of patients seen, complexity of cases, stopping surgery, etc.). Excessive workload can lead to burnout particularly quickly in older physicians. Work barriers should be minimized, and ageist stereotypes should be resisted. It is also helpful for organizations to offer retirement education and guidance, including access to financial advice. Organizations also are served well by creation of post-retirement opportunities including peer support, teaching, mentoring, administration and other non-clinical activities. This approach maintains access for younger physicians, patients and administrators to the experience and wisdom of older physicians. Organizations should avoid mandatory retirement ages; and they also must recognize the limits of cognitive testing administered for the first time to older physicians.[3] Organizations that address these issues are not just being altruistic. They are responsible for many challenges associated with retirement including patient care continuity, maintenance of deserved reputations for expertise, and succession of physicians in the institution/hospital. Planning to manage these issues prospectively is far preferable to managing them emergently when key physicians leave.

Many other challenges accompany retirement including maintenance of a physician's identity, interactions with a spouse, activities to fill the days (as much as desired and needed), long-term financial security (to the point at which the retired physician does not have to worry about money constantly) and others. Most physicians who retire and say that "it was a mistake" might have had a better experience if planning and support had been more thoughtful; and they might have continued to contribute to medical practice and patient care quality longer on a part-time basis than they did if organizational support, opportunities and intervention had been utilized. Many physicians who are thriving in "retirement" are happily as busy as they ever were, but with more control over their schedules. Many successful physicians are Type A people and have high Grit scores! They would be unhappy and feel useless doing nothing; but when they recognize what makes them happy and fill their post-medical days with those activities and friends, then their "retirements" are successful. I have trouble thinking of people involved in so many activities as retired just because they are not seeing patients. Rather, I regard them as having **transitioned** into the next phase of their productive lives.

Retiring too late creates obvious problems such as an increased number of justified malpractice suits. However, retiring too early can be similarly damaging to society and the physician, although metrics might be less obvious. Everyone in medicine (regardless of our current age) should give considerable thought to this complex issue. It affects us all.

References

1. Hirschbein LD. William Osler and the fixed period: conflicting medical and popular ideas about old age. *Arch Intern Med* 2001;161(17):2074–8.
2. Adler RG, Constantinou C. Knowing – or not knowing – when to stop: cognitive decline in ageing doctors. *Med J Aust* 2008;189(11–12):622–4.
3. Sataloff RT. The aging physician and surgeon. *Ear Nose Throat J* 2016;95(4–5):E35.
4. Eva KW, Cunnington JP. The difficulty with experience: does practice increase susceptibility to premature closure? *J Contin Educ Health Prof* 2006;26(3):192–8.
5. Caulford PG, Lamb SB, Kaigas TB, Hanna E, Norman GR, David DA. Physician incompetence: specific problems and predictors. *Acad Med* 1994;69(10 Suppl):S16–8.
6. Bieliauskas LA, Langenecker SA, Graver CJ, Lee HJ, O'Neill JS, Greenfield LJ. Cognitive changes and retirement among senior surgeons: Results from the CCRASS study. *J Am Coll Surg* 2008;207:69–79.

7. "USC Gerontology." *Master's Degree in Gerontology Online*, gerontology.usc.edu/resources/infographics/americans-are-living-longer/. Accessed 16 Jan. 2019.
8. Silver MP, Hamilton AD, Biswas A, Warrick NI. A systemic review of physician retirement planning. *Human Resources for Health* 2016;14:67.
9. American Academy of Otolaryngology – Head and Neck Surgery. Socioeconomic survey: National trends. *Bulletin* 2018;37(4).
10. McGuirt Jr WF, McGuirt Sr WF. Otolaryngology Retirement Profile in the Southeastern United States. *Laryngoscope* 2002;112:213–215.
11. Collier R. Diagnosing the aging physician. *CMAJ* 2008;178(9):1121–3.
12. Petersen RC. Clinical practice. Mild cognitive impairment. *N Engl J Med* 2011;364(23):2227–34.
13. Alzheimer's Association. 2009 Alzheimer's disease facts and figures. *Alzheimers Dement* 2009;5(3):234–70.

Reprinted with modifications by permission of SAGE Publications, Inc. from:
   Sataloff RT. Physicians and Retirement. *ENT J*; in press

About the Author

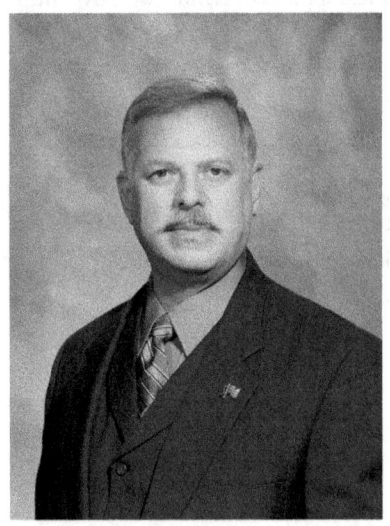

Robert T. Sataloff, M.D., D.M.A., F.A.C.S. is Professor and Chairman, Department of Otolaryngology-Head and Neck Surgery and Senior Associate Dean for Clinical Academic Specialties, Drexel University College of Medicine. He is also Adjunct Professor in the department of Otolaryngology–Head and Neck Surgery at Thomas Jefferson University, as well as Adjunct Clinical Professor at Temple University and the Philadelphia College of Osteopathic Medicine; and he is on the faculty of the Academy of Vocal Arts. He serves as Conductor of the Thomas Jefferson University Choir. Dr. Sataloff is also a professional singer and singing teacher. He holds an undergraduate degree from Haverford College in Music Theory and Composition; graduated from Jefferson Medical College, Thomas Jefferson University; received a Doctor of Musical Arts in Voice Performance from Combs College of Music; and he completed Residency in Otolaryngology-Head and Neck Surgery and a Fellowship in Otology, Neurotology and Skull Base Surgery at the University of Michigan. Dr. Sataloff is Chairman of the Boards of Directors of the Voice Foundation and of the American Institute for Voice and Ear Research. He also has served as Chairman of the Board of Governors of Graduate Hospital; President of the American Laryngological Association, the International Association of Phonosurgery, the Pennsylvania Academy of Otolaryngology–Head and Neck Surgery, and The American Society of Geriatric Otolaryngology, and in numerous other leadership positions. Dr. Sataloff is Editor-in-Chief of the *Journal of Voice*; Editor-in-Chief of *Ear, Nose and Throat Journal*; Associate Editor of the *Journal of Singing*, and on the editorial boards of numerous otolaryngology journals. He has written over 1,000 publications, including 65 books, and he has been awarded more than $5 million in research funding. He has invented more than 75 laryngeal microsurgical instruments distributed currently by Integra Medical, ossicular replacement prostheses produced by Grace Medical, and novel laryngeal prostheses with Boston Medical. His medical practice is limited to care of the professional voice and to otology. Dr. Sataloff has developed numerous novel surgical procedures including total temporal bone resection for formerly untreatable skull base malignancy, laryngeal microflap and mini-microflap procedures, vocal fold lipoinjection, vocal fold lipoimplantation, and others. Dr. Sataloff is recognized as one of the founders of the field of voice, having written the first modern comprehensive article on care of singers, and the first chapter and book on care of the professional voice, as well as having influenced the evolution of the field through his own efforts and through the Voice Foundation for nearly 4 decades. Dr. Sataloff has been recognized by Best Doctors in America (Woodward White Athens) every year since 1992, *Philadelphia Magazine* since 1997, and Castle Connolly's 'America's Top Doctors' since 2002.

Index

AAMC *see* Association of American Medical Colleges
AAN *see* American Academy of Neurology
AAO-H&NS *see* American Academy of Otolaryngology-Head and Neck Surgery
AAO-HNSF *see* American Academy of Otolaryngology-Head and Neck Surgery Foundation
ABEA *see* American BronchoEsophalogical Association
Academic practice 3–4, 7, 9, 18, 30
Academy of Doctors of Audiology 173
Accountable care organizations (ACOs) 108
Accreditation Council for Graduate Medical Education 7
ACO *see* Accountable care organizations (ACOs)
ACS *see* American College of Surgeons
ACS NSQIP *see* American College of Surgeons National Quality Improvement Program (ACS NSQIP)
ADEA *see* Age Discrimination in Employment Act Age Discrimination in Employment Act (ADEA) 221, 224
Age discrimination 221–2, 224
Agency for Health Care Research 97
Aging 49, 218–40, 252–4
ALA *see* American Laryngological Association American Academy of Audiology 173
American Academy of Neurology 100
American Academy of Otolaryngology - Speech, Voice and Swallowing Committee 49
American Academy of Otolaryngology-Head and Neck Surgery 57–8, 99, 103, 105–6, 111, 128, 179, 190, 207
American Academy of Otolaryngology-Head and Neck Surgery Foundation (AAO-HNSF) 106, 105

INDEX

American Board of Medical Specialties 31, 256
American Board of Otolaryngology 106, 180
American Bronchoesophalogical Association 47
American College of Graduate Medical Education 31
American College of Surgeons (ACS) 19, 96, 109, 113, 208, 223, 228, 249, 251, 256
  Board of Governors Committee on Physician Competency and Health 228
  Clinical Congress 2246–7
American College of Surgeons Board of Governors Committee on Physician Competency and Health 228
American Laryngological Association 43, 49, 57, 259
American Medical Association 156, 183, 190
American Society of Anesthesiologists 108
Andrea, M. 58
Arts medicine 34–6, 40–1, 52–3
Association of American Medical Colleges 7, 68, 179
Audiologist 11, 28, 172–3, 177–8
Audiology *see* Hearing
Behavior
  Disruptive behaviors 183–5
  Inappropriate language 184
  Physical intimidation 184
  Sexually inappropriate behavior 183–4
Big data 111–4 Billing 97, 142, 152–4

Board of Directors 159–62, 180
British Medical Journal Open 258
Case reports 13, 80, 135–6
Catholic University of America 232
CCRASS Study (cognitive changes and retirement among senior surgeons) 226–7, 238–9
Centers for Disease Control and Prevention 100
Centers for Medicare and Medicaid Services 96, 105
Centralized Otolaryngology Research Efforts (CORE) 91, 128, 103–4
Certification 6, 31, 67, 69, 106, 173, 223–4, 238, 256
CLD *see* Lyme disease
Clinical education and training 30, 43–53, 68–70
Clinical practice
  Clinical guidelines 52, 99–102, 113, 156–7, 187, 209, 228, 256
  Outcomes 13, 20–1, 41, 47–52, 74, 76, 79, 82, 84, 108–9, 111–3, 160, 204, 208, 212, 215, 219, 222, 226, 238–9, 256–7
  Scope of practice 22–3, 172–5, 177
Clinical research 4, 9–12, 46, 49–50, 74–6, 87, 128, 148
Clinical trials 78–9, 82, 84–5, 87–9, 94–5, 135, 212–6
CMS *see* Centers for Medicare and Medicaid Services
Combined Otolaryngology Spring Meeting (COSM) 128
Congress *see* U.S. Congress
Consolidated Standards of Reporting Trials (CONSORT) 84, 94–5

CONSORT *see* Consolidated Standards of Reporting Trials
Consortia 60–1
Continuing education 256
CORE *see* Centralized Otolaryngology Research Efforts Correction (of published papers)
COSM *see* Combined Otolaryngology Spring Meeting
Cosmetic surgery 30, 188, 254
Cossman, D. 146–8
Cross-sectional studies 222
Dana, J. 65
Data science 112–14
Dean's Tax 3
Demonstroscope *see* Lukens' demonstroscope
Direct-to-consumer advertising 90–2
Doctors
   Young Doctors 67–70
Drexel University College of Medicine 7, 26
Drugs 85, 87, 106, 198
   Abuse 223
   Investigational New Drug Application 87–8
   Marketing and promotion 88, 90–3
   Research and development 11, 87–9
   Risk factors 80, 84–5, 87–8, 96–7
   Trials 88, 99
DTCA *see* Direct-to-consumer advertising (DTCA)
Ear, Nose & Throat Journal 114, 117–8, 173, 206
Eberlein, T.J. 129
EBM *see* Evidence-based medicine
Editorial board 14, 16, 120, 123–6, 133, 180–1

Education
   Affiliates and multiple sites 13, 18, 26, 28, 31, 35, 44–5, 68, 70, 76, 225
   Curriculum 6–7, 28, 31, 44–5, 49, 68–70
   Medical education 4, 6–7, 20, 28, 31–2, 35, 43–5, 54, 68, 70, 76, 225
   Student education 7–8, 11–12, 19–21, 27, 29–31, 44–5, 48, 50–1, 70, 123, 126, 130–1, 200, 204
Elsberg, L. *see also* American Laryngological Association 43–5, 54
Elsevier 133–4
Emergency Medical Treatment and Active Labor Act (EMTALA) 150
Emotional intelligence 192 Employee Retirement Income Security Act (ERISA) 173
EMTALA *see* Emergency Medical Treatment and Active Labor Act
Endoscopy 52, 131, 172
European Laryngological Association 57
Evidence-based medicine (EBM) 78, 81, 111, 135, 191
Excerpta Medica 134
Expert witness 255–7
FAA *see* Federal Aviation Administration
Facebook 112
Faculty 3–7, 10–11, 26–8, 52, 65, 75, 130, 165, 201
FDA *see* U.S. Food and Drug Administration

INDEX

Federal Aviation Administration (FAA) 221, 224, 228, 233
Federal Bureau of Investigation (FBI) 221, 223
Federal Code of Regulations (32 CFR 219.102 [D]). 96
Federal law *see* Legislation - Federal law
Federation of State Medical Boards 224
Gender 154, 182
    Salary discrepancy 181–2
    Women in Otolaryngology (WIO) 179–81
Geriatrics 174, 207–10, 219, 229
Google 113
Gould, W.J. 47, 52
Graduate Education Foundation 27–8
Graffman, G. 41
Guardian, The (Newspaper) 258
Guides to the Evaluation of Permanent Impairment 189–93
Hammerbacher, J. 126
Harris, T.J. 45
Harvard Medical School 62, 204
Health Care Quality Improvement Act 184–5
Health Information Technology for Economic and Clinical Health Act (HITECH) 113
Health insurance 74–6, 96, 108, 139–42, 144–6, 149–50, 152–4, 173, 228
Health Insurance Portability and Accountability Act of 1996 (HIPAA) 74–6, 97
Healthcare Costs 69, 74–6, 89, 97, 109–9, 141, 145–6, 213–16
Hearing
Hearing aids 172–4, 177–8, 187
Hearing loss 26, 146, 187–8
    Occupational hearing loss 189–93
HIPAA *see* Health Insurance Portability and Accountability Act
Hippocratic Oath 32, 38
Hirano, M. 47, 52
HITECH *see* Health Information Technology for Economic and Clinical Health Act
Hofstra North Shore-Long Island Jewish School of Medicine 69
House of Representatatives 169–70
Human subjects research *see* Research - Human subjects research
ICF *see* International Classification of Functioning, Disability and Health
ICSOM *see* International Conference of Symphony and Opera Musicians
IDSA *see* Infectious Diseases Society of America
Impact factor *see* Publishing - Impact factor
IND *see* Drugs - Investigational New Drug
Indexing 11–12, 15, 136
    Index Medicus 12, 15
    Institute for Scientific Information 12, 15
    Scopus 15
Index Medicus *see* Indexing
Infectious Diseases Society of America 100
Institute for Scientific Information *see* Indexing
Institutional Review Board 11, 74, 85, 89, 96–8

Interdisciplinary medicine 32–6, 40, 43, 47–8, 53, 249, 251
Interdisciplinary teams 9–10, 19, 30–3, 48, 51, 87, 108–9, 176, 200, 221, 239–41
International Arts Medicine Association *see also* Arts Medicine 34
International Classification of Functioning, Disability and Health (ICF) 191
International Committee of Medical Journal Editors 84–5
International Conference of Symphony and Opera Musicians 40
Interview 60–1, 65–7, 195
Research interviews 80, 228
Investigational New Drugs *see* Drugs
Ioannidis, J. 81–2
IRB *see* Institutional Review Board
Isshiki, N. 52
JACS *see* Journal of the American College of Surgeons
Jadad *see also* Randomized, controlled trials 94–5
JAMA *see* Journal of the American Medical Association
Jefferson Medical College 69, 180
Johns, M. 58
Journal of the American College of Surgeons 128–9
Journal of Voice 120, 124–5, 133
Journals *see* Publishing - Journals
Knight, F. 44–5
Krouse, J. 125
Laryngeal electromyography *see* Laryngology - Measurement and assessment instruments
Laryngeal mirror 41, 46
Laryngology
Anatomy and physiology 36, 45, 47, 49–52
Assessment and diagnosis 47–52
Laryngeal framework surgery 52
Measurement and assessment tools 44–47, 51, 143, 214
Neuroanatomy and neurophysiology 50
Neurolaryngology 49–50
Laryngoscope *see also* Laryngology - Measurement and assessment tools 44–5, 47
Legislation
Copyright law 16
Discrimination 219–24
Federal law 146, 149–55, 167, 169–71, 222, 240, 242
Letters to the Editor 119, 128
Level of evidence *see also* Evidence-based medicine 79, 101
Liability 155–7, 159–60, 173, 214, 229–30
LinkedIn 112
Lipschultz, J. 114
Literature review 8, 11–13, 50, 74, 77–80, 87, 89, 94–5, 99, 101, 124–30, 133, 135–6, 219–20, 232, 234, 239
LOE *see* Level of evidence
Lukens' demonstroscope 46
Lyme disease 100
Magnetic Resonance Imaging (MRI) 146
Malpractice 32, 142, 150, 155–7, 163, 174, 227–8, 255–7
Massachusetts Eye and Ear Infirmary 62

INDEX

Massachusetts General Hospital 204, 213
Mayo Clinic 46, 69–70
MCAT *see* Medical college admission test
McKinnon, B. 81, 113
Medicaid 96, 105, 108, 140
Medical college admission test 70
Medical Librarian 11
Medical record 9, 13, 74, 76, 106, 163, 204
Medicare 96–7, 105, 149–154, 173, 222, 224, 227
MEDLINE 45, 219
Merck & Co., Inc 134
Merit-Based Incentive Payment System 106
Meta-analyses 79–82
Moore, P. 46
MRI *see* Magnetic Resonance Imaging
National Institute on Deafness and Other Communication Disorders 186
National Institutes of Health 87, 100, 103–4
Medical Musings 280
National Practitioner Data Bank 184
National Resident Matching Program 60, 180
Neurolaryngology *see* Laryngology - Neurolaryngology
Neurological disorders 15, 34, 48, 229, 237
Neuropsychology 220, 222, 226, 229, 233–4, 237, 239
Neurosurgery 15, 33–4, 212, 249
Neurotology 29–31, 33–4, 50, 146, 214
New York Times 65, 227

NIDCD *see* National Institute on Deafness and Other Communication Disorders
Obamacare 139–40, 149
Occupational hearing loss *see* Hearing loss - Occupational hearing loss
OREBM *see* Outcomes Research and Evidence-Based Medicine Committee
Organ harvesting 258–60
ORL-H&NS *see* Otolaryngology-Head & Neck Surgery
Orthopedic surgery 217
Ossof, R 53
Otolaryngology *see* Otolaryngology-Head & Neck Surgery
Otolaryngology-Head & Neck Surgery 3, 25–31, 34, 43, 45–52, 57–63, 76, 95, 99, 103–6, 111, 125, 128, 165, 168, 179–82, 190–2, 200–11, 207, 215, 253
Outcomes Research and Evidence-Based Medicine Committee *see also* Evidence-based medicine 111
Osler, Sir W. 261
Patient Protection and Affordable Care Act (PPACA) 148, 155
Patient safety 19–24, 74, 156, 169, 172, 178, 229–30, 238, 257
Patil, D.J. 112–3
Peer review *see* Publishing - Peer review
Pennsylvania Medical Society 153
Pennsylvania Medical Society v. Marconis 153
Pennsylvania State College of Medicine 69
Performance measures 106
Performing arts *see* Arts medicine

Performing arts medicine *see* Arts medicine
Pharmaceuticals 87–93, 134
Physical Therapist 11, 33
Physician
    Aging 210–38, 261
    Competency 5, 27, 43, 68, 210–11, 214–7, 219–226, 230
    Retirement 173, 201, 210–13, 216–21, 224–30, 261–5
    Shortage 190–2, 210, 220
    Well-being 186–7, 196
    Physician Quality Reporting System 105
Physicians' political action committee *see* Politics - Physicians' political action committee
Plagiarism 121, 127
Pocket veto 170
Politics 5, 7, 13, 65, 95–8, 118, 128, 131–4, 143–5, 148, 156–62, 164–5
    Physicians' political action committee 165
PPACA *see* Patient Protection and Affordable Care Act
Practice parameters 95–7, 151
Price control 146–8
Protocol Registration System (PRS) 85
PRS *see* Protocol Registration System
Publishing
    As a teaching tool 124–6
    Bias 16–17, 101, 118, 127, 133–4
    Conflict of interest 100, 124, 133–4, 160–2
    Editorial Board 14–17, 78, 80, 84, 112–4, 117–23, 127–30, 133, 135, 180–2
    Ethics 13, 16, 85, 117–8, 121–3, 127–9, 258–60
    Impact factor 94, 136
    Journals 6, 9–15, 74, 78, 80–1, 90–1, 110, 112–28, 130, 172–3
    Peer review 12–17, 74, 78–82, 94, 118–22, 127–9, 133–6, 220–2, 252, 257
Publishing Research Consortium 17, 121
PubMed 219
QCDR *see* Qualified Clinical Data Registries
Qualified Clinical Data Registries (QCDR) 105
Quality improvement project 96–8, 106, 109, 184, 222
Quaternary care 108–9
Randomized trials 74, 79, 82, 94–5, 212, 214
Reflux 51
Reg-ent 105–6
Reimbursement 96, 105, 145, 149, 152, 163, 181, 187, 214
Research
    Bias 79, 82–3, 100–1, 114, 205
    Human subjects research 7, 11, 84, 87–8, 96–8
    Research team 11, 112
Residents
    Application for 60–4
    Education and training 3–4, 6–22, 25–30, 35, 45–54, 70, 75–6, 123–20, 123–6, 130–1, 149, 180–1, 194–5, 225–6
    Hours 19–24
    Well-being 192–4, 204
Rogers, W. 258

Rosen, C. 58
Rubin, A. 58
Sataloff, J. 188
Schmalbach, C. 125
Scope of practice *see* Clinical practice - Scope of practice
Senate *see* U.S. Senate
Shoulder injury related to vaccine administration (SIRVA) 197–9
Sidney Kimmel Medical College *see also* Thomas Jefferson University 69
Sinai Hospital 229
Singing *see* Arts medicine
Singing teacher 35–6, 46–7, 53
SIRVA *see* Shoulder injury related to vaccine administration
Skillern, R.H. 45
Smith, L. 58
Speech-Language Pathology 11, 35–6, 41, 51–3, 57, 59, 249
Statistics 8, 11–12, 82, 91, 94, 98, 109, 112–4, 120, 128, 130, 187
Stem cell 253
Sundberg, J. 58
Surgery (General) *see also* Otolaryngology-Head & Neck surgery; Neurosurgery, Cosmetic surgery 15, 17, 23, 25, 108, 145, 180, 204, 223–6, 229, 232, 251
Surgery
   Ethics 258–60
   Geriatric surgery 173, 207–10, 229
   Adverse events 204–6, 208
   Televised 46–7
   Transplantation 258–60
Surgical Care Improvement Project 96
Swallowing disorders 45–7, 166
Tardy, M.E. 46–7

Teamwork *see* Interdiciplinary teams
Telemedicine 109, 211–16
The Joint Commission 7, 184, 256
Thomas Jefferson University 69, 180
Thyroid 51, 128–9
Tinnitus 186
Tort 155–8
Transplantation *see* Surgery - Transplantation
Trustees 160–2
U.S. Congress 21, 159, 167, 169–70, 221
U.S. Department of Health and Human Services 155
U.S. Food and Drug Administration Office of Prescription Drug Promotion
U.S. Senate 169–70
UHC *see* United Healthcare UHG *see* UnitedHealth Group
United States Secretary of Health and Human Services 153
UnitedHealth Group (UHG) 173
UnitedHealthcare (UHC) 173
University of Michigan 3, 47, 62, 226
University of Texas 66
University of Virginia 108, 229
VA *see* Veterans Administration
Veterans Administration 141–2
Veterans Integrated Service Networks (VISN) 141
Videoconferencing 26–7, 212–13
VISN *see* Veterans Integrated Service Networks
Voice and voice disorders 29, 35–8, 41–53, 128–9, 131, 172, 214, 249
Voice coach 41
Voice Foundation 47, 57–8

von Leden, H. 46–7, 52
Wilders, J.S. 44
WIO *see* Gender - Women in Otolaryngology
Women in Otolaryngology *see* Gender - Women in Otolaryngology

Women's Medical College 180
World Health Assembly 191
World Health Organization 57, 191
World Voice Day 57–9